YMCA Fitness Testing and Assessment Manual

Fourth Edition

YMCA of the USA

Lawrence A. Golding, PhD, Editor

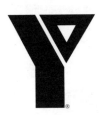

Library of Congress Cataloging-in-Publication Data

YMCA fitness testing and assessment manual / YMCA of the USA--4th ed.
   p. cm.
  Rev. ed of Y's way to physical fitness.
  Includes bibliographical references and index.
  ISBN 0-7360-3316-5
   1. Physical fitness. 2. Physical fitness--Testing. 3. Exercise. I. YMCA of the USA. II.
  Y's way to physical fitness.

GV481.Y46 2000
613.7--dc21

                                                           00-038310

ISBN: 0-7360-3316-5

Published for the YMCA of the USA by Human Kinetics Publishers, Inc.
Copyright © 2000 by National Council of Young Men's Christian Associations of the United States of America

This book is a revised edition of *Y's Way to Physical Fitness, Third Edition,* published in 1989 by Human Kinetics Publishers, Inc.

YMCA Project Coordinator: Michael Spezzano
Editor: Lawrence A. Golding, PhD
Acquisitions Editor: Patricia Sammann
Managing Editor: Leigh LaHood
Copyeditor: Amie Bell
Proofreader: Myla Smith
Indexer: Betty Frizzéll
Permission Manager: Cheri Banks
Graphic Designer: Fred Starbird
Graphic Artists: Francine Hamerski, Dawn Sills
Cover Designer: Keith Blomberg
Photographers (interior): Photos on pages 3, 7, 15, 49, 87, and 159 courtesy of the YMCA of the USA. Photos on pages 107, 149, 156, and 167 by Tom Roberts. Photos on pages 113, 133-135, and 146 from YMCA, 1989, *Y's Way to Physical Fitness,* 3rd ed. (Champaign, IL: Human Kinetics).
Illustrators: All figures in chapter 3 courtesy of the YMCA, except figure 3.19 by Marie T. Dauenheimer. Figures 4.1-4.9, 4.11-4.20, 4.22-4.25, 5.1-5.4, and 6.18, and tables 6.1 and 6.2 by Mic Greenberg. Figures 6.20 and 6.21 courtesy of Lawrence A. Golding.
Printer: Versa Press

Printed in the United States of America   10 9 8 7 6 5 4 3 2 1

Copies of this book may be purchased from the YMCA Program Store, P.O. Box 5076, Champaign, IL 61825-5076, 800-747-0089.

The YMCA of the USA does not operate or manage any health and fitness programs or facilities.

Contents

Preface

The primary purpose of *YMCA Fitness Testing and Assessment Manual* is to present information on how to administer the YMCA Fitness Assessment protocol. Included is the standard testing protocol, national norm tables for adults, and the rationale behind the various tests. This book is the course text for the YMCA Fitness Specialist training course, but students, staff, and volunteers who desire to learn how to administer the YMCA fitness tests will also find it useful. This testing program has been used successfully for nearly 30 years and is one of the most reliable and valid test batteries for adult physical fitness testing.

This book evolved from the text *Y's Way to Physical Fitness*, which was first published in 1973 and revised in 1982 and again in 1989. *Y's Way to Physical Fitness* was designed to enable the local YMCA fitness director to organize and administer physical fitness testing, understand the basic exercise physiology of the test battery, and conduct the YMCA physical fitness test battery and be able to interpret the test results for the participant.

The majority of the testing and assessment material from *Y's Way to Physical Fitness* is still viable. This new book incorporates that information along with updates to the testing protocol and new norms, the best adult fitness norms available anywhere. In addition, chapters on anatomy, physiology, and kinesiology help readers to better understand and interpret the test battery. These chapters provide valuable information, particularly to readers taking the YMCA of the USA Fitness Specialist training and certification course.

The book is divided into three parts:

- The YMCA and fitness
- Basics of anatomy, physiology, and kinesiology
- Fitness testing at the YMCA

Part I includes chapter 1, which describes the history of the Y's Way to Physical Fitness program and materials, and chapter 2, which discusses the YMCA's program objectives and the YMCA Health and Fitness program and training structure. Part II covers the basics of anatomy, physiology, and kinesiology. Chapter 3 describes muscular structure, and chapter 4 focuses on the cardiorespiratory system. Finally, part III includes an introduction to fitness testing in chapter 5 and descriptions of the administration of each of the tests in the YMCA Fitness Assessment protocol in chapter 6. Chapter 7 offers the fitness director guidelines for organizing and conducting fitness testing. The sidebars throughout part III provide basic information on using YMCA Fitness Analyst software as part of a fitness testing program.

The appendixes provide additional materials for fitness directors to use in their testing programs. Appendix A contains sample health screening, medical clearance, and informed consent forms. Appendix B has masters for scoring sheets for all YMCA fitness tests. Appendix C provides basic information on using YMCA Fitness Analyst software in a testing program, and appendix D is a list of common activities and the number of calories burned per minute during those activities.

The YMCA of the USA pioneered fitness testing back in the 1960s, first published *Y's Way to Physical Fitness* in the early 1970s, and continues today to improve and update the testing process. With this new text we hope to continue this long tradition, helping fitness directors to give YMCA members the guidance and motivation they need to get fit and stay fit.

Acknowledgments

The first edition of *Y's Way to Physical Fitness*, the source for much of the information in this current manual, was compiled from the input of 50 individuals who are or were leaders in exercise physiology, sports medicine, and physical fitness.

Much of the work of this group is still contained in this manual. Here is a list of the original research and writing team:

Donald C. Bingham
George Burger
L. Eugene Cantrall
James Chapel
Kenneth Cooper, MD
David L. Costill, PhD
Paul Couzelis, PhD
Thomas K. Cureton, PhD
William C. Day, PhD
Belvin Doane, PhD
David W. Dunsworth
Delmar Eggert
Charles Eising
Donald S. Fletcher
Rueben B. Frost, PhD
Emery Gay
John F. Gibbs
Warren Giese, PhD
John Gillingham
Lawrence A. Golding, PhD
M.F. Graham, MD
Russell Harris
Tom Harris
William L. Haskell, PhD
James Havlick

Gordon E. Hendrickson
Bernard Howes, DDS
Alfred K. Johnson
Jack J. Joseph, EdD
Robert Jurci
Ken Kendro
Russell Kisby
Robert L. McFarland, PhD
Roger Martin
Alexander Melleby
Clayton A. Myers, PhD
Francis J. O'Brien, DMD
Wes Ogle
Arne Olson, PhD
Stan Pedzick
Michael L. Pollock, PhD
Wayne Ray
Paul M. Ribisl, PhD
Robert Salisbury
Charles H. Shattuck, Jr.
Wayne Sinning, PhD
James Skinner, PhD
Jack H. Wilmore, PhD
Michael S. Yuhasz, PhD

The volunteers who served on the YMCA Health Enhancement Advisory Committee during the developmental period of the first edition include the following:

E. Stanley Enlund
Samuel Fox III, MD
Gary A. Fry, MD
Lawrence A. Golding, PhD

Clayton R. Myers, PhD
Nanette K. Wenger, MD
Jack H. Wilmore, PhD

From the day the book was published, the editors realized that it would need to be not only revised but also rewritten to include the many women involved in YMCA programs and to add new national programs. With the help of many individuals and committees, the first edition was revised. Virtually all physical directors who have ever attended certification workshops, and certainly the workshop faculties, provided ideas and suggestions for the revision—some formally, some informally, some written, some verbal. Some of the major contributors to the second edition, especially those on formal committees, are listed here:

Nancy Albertson
Merve Bennett
Jeff Boone
Sam Brown
Joni Coe
Rich Escutia
Ron Fish
Herman Gohn
Glenn Gress
Andrew Jackson, PhD
Larry Johnson
John Joyce
Dave King
Phil Mallers
Dan Ochs
Pat Owens

Dennis Palmer
Sharon Plowman, PhD
Terrell K. Puffer
Jackie Puhl, PhD
Kent Rea
Ed Reeves
Pat Ryan
Jeff Sadowsky
Jim Scott
Jim Seidl
Neil Sol, PhD
Michael Thompson
Pat Thornton
Steve Totten
Dick Webster
William B. Zuti, PhD

Although the membership of the YMCA Health Enhancement Advisory Committee changed through the ensuing years, the committee encouraged the revision. Dr. William Zuti, who became the new director of the National Health Enhancement Program in 1980, helped to facilitate its completion. The members of the committee in 1981 should be recognized for their contributions:

Samuel Fox III, MD
Lawrence A. Golding, PhD
William G. Hettler, MD
Charles A. Pinderhughes, MD

Michael L. Pollock, PhD
Jesse L. Steinfeld, MD
William B. Zuti, PhD

The third edition, published in 1989, was not a revision in the strictest sense; instead, it was more of an updating and streamlining. The major revision was the new norms, which reflected six age categories for each sex. These norms are the most extensive on the adult population in the United States. We want to give a special thank you to Anne Lindsay, who did most of the work in collecting raw data for the new norms, and to Kirk Golding, who did the computer programming. Anne is a former YMCA physical director who did her graduate work in exercise physiology at the University of Nevada at Las Vegas. Kirk Golding helped Cardinal Health Systems to develop the original software for the Y's Way to Physical Fitness program.

In addition to the new norms, the body composition prediction formulas used for determining percent body fat and target weight were made uniform for both men and women. Each uses the same three or four skinfold measurement sites.

Questionnaires were sent to YMCA physical directors so they could give input on needed changes in the revision. In addition, in 1986 a committee was formed comprising Physical Fitness Specialists' Workshop directors and their physiology consultants. This group added to the third edition. The members of this group are the following:

George Babish
Tom Burke, EdD
Lawrence A. Golding, PhD
Mike Heilbronn
Prescott Johnson, PhD
Dick Jones
Stephen Kaye
Alice Kazanowski, PhD
Cliff Lothery

Powell McClellan, PhD
Dan Ochs
Gary Pechar, PhD
Steve Siconolfi, PhD
Wayne Sinning, PhD
Pat Thornton
John Usmial
Anthony Whitney, PhD

As this latest edition is published in 2000, we want to make special mention of the work of the three editors of the first three editions of *Y's Way to Physical Fitness*: Lawrence A. Golding, Clayton A. Myers, and Wayne E. Sinning. These individuals spent countless hours reviewing, organizing, and editing all of the material contained in the original texts. Without their selfless volunteer efforts and dedication, the fitness testing program of the YMCA would not exist. They are true pioneers in the physical fitness movement in America, and they have contributed invaluably to every YMCA in the United States.

The YMCA of the USA would like to acknowledge the editor of this text, Lawrence A. Golding, PhD, FACSM, University of Nevada, Las Vegas. For 30 years, Larry has consistently given passionate leadership to the YMCA Physical Fitness Testing program as a volunteer. Not only was he instrumental in developing the initial protocol, but he also has been intimately involved with all of the subsequent revisions, the ongoing training of YMCA staff, and the processing and storing of fitness test data. His commitment to YMCA Health and Fitness is unequaled.

The development process to update the manual into its present form was led by Michael J. Spezzano, YMCA of the USA Associate Director of Program Development, whose primary responsibility is for health and fitness programs.

In many ways, this manual is the cornerstone of physical fitness in the YMCA. Many individuals have been responsible for the development and ongoing revision of this material, too many to list them all here. The YMCA Fitness Testing and Assessment protocol represents a true YMCA grass-roots effort. It was conceived, developed, and revised by the users, the staff, and the volunteers who administer it daily. This book is dedicated to you.

Part I

The YMCA and Fitness

Chapter 1

Introduction to YMCA Fitness Testing

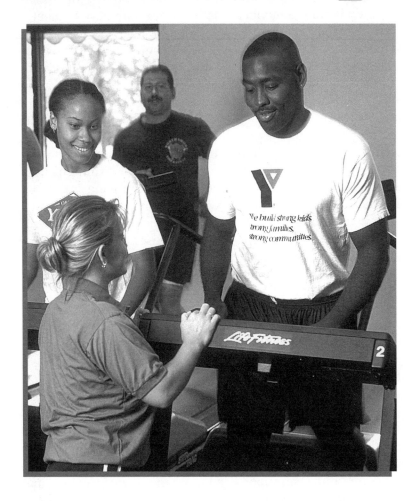

The history of the YMCA Fitness Testing and Assessment Program is an interesting study of both the fitness movement in the United States and the YMCA's response to it. As physical fitness exploded as a national pastime in the 1960s and 1970s, the YMCA responded by developing a nationwide plan for physical fitness, which included a standardized fitness testing protocol. Fifty experts in physical fitness, exercise physiology, and sports medicine drafted the first proposed national fitness testing protocol and program and presented it to the National YMCA in 1971. Called the "Y's Way to Physical Fitness," this test battery reflected the most up-to-date scientific information and had the following advantages:

1. It was simple to administer and interpret.
2. It required a minimum of equipment.

3. It required little time to administer.

4. It was within the YMCA fitness director's capabilities.

5. It reflected changes in the fitness parameters that were emphasized in most YMCA fitness classes.

6. It was safe when administered according to the established protocols.

In 1973 the first edition of *Y's Way to Physical Fitness* was published. Training and certification courses were instituted to standardize the administration of the fitness tests. The grass-roots impetus behind the Y's Way to Physical Fitness Program involved many people, and it became a model for national program development.

Almost immediately after publication of *Y's Way to Physical Fitness*, the need to revise the book became evident. Other YMCA fitness programs were developing, such as weight management, back exercise, and cardiac rehabilitation, and YMCA fitness programs were enrolling an increasing number of women. Physical fitness programs at the YMCA were growing exponentially. In 1975 a national advisory board was appointed, and a director of the National YMCA Cardiovascular Program was named to oversee all of the new fitness programs.

In the years following the publication of the first edition, hundreds of people became involved in the revision of *Y's Way to Physical Fitness*. During this time the national program changed its name to the YMCA Health Enhancement Program. The national headquarters moved from New York City to Chicago, and a new director of Health Enhancement Programs was appointed. The second edition of *Y's Way to Physical Fitness* was completed and released in 1982.

As YMCA fitness programs continued to grow and diversify during the 1980s, the population became more fit and new resources became available. This trend led to the decision to develop a third edition of *Y's Way to Physical Fitness*. The third edition was released in 1989 and included new norms for all tests based on the results from approximately 20,000 participants. For the first time the norms were divided into six age groups for both men and women. Specific modifications to the testing protocol included new workload settings for the bicycle ergometer tests and use of the same skinfold sites for both men and women.

By the late 1990s, it became clear that the format and premise of *Y's Way to Physical Fitness* needed to be updated. The text was designed originally to be a complete resource not only for testing and evaluation but also for conducting physical fitness programs; yet YMCA health and fitness programs had evolved far beyond what was contained in the text. The materials in new YMCA textbooks for a number of health and fitness programs had superceded much of the program information in *Y's Way to Physical Fitness*. In addition, the certification process in the YMCA of the USA had expanded with several new health and fitness certifications. The majority of the physical fitness test protocol contained in the original text, however, was still valid and useful. This manual retains that protocol, with two major changes that were introduced in 1997: a new half sit-up test to measure muscle strength and endurance, replacing the full sit-up test, and updated norm tables based on the results of 35,000 fitness tests conducted at local YMCAs.

Training Courses

After *Y's Way to Physical Fitness* was first published, the YMCA of the USA developed a Fitness Specialist training course to review the physiological principles on which the various test battery items were based and to train individuals in the correct protocols for the YMCA tests. Certification as a YMCA Fitness Specialist confirmed that an individual had attended the five-day training course, knew how to administer the test battery, and could validly interpret the results to YMCA members.

Ten to 15 YMCA Fitness Specialist training courses have been held each year for the past 25 years, resulting in approximately 8,000 certified YMCA Fitness Specialists. Although the majority of these individuals were staff and volunteers from local YMCAs, participants also included personnel from other fitness organizations and centers, police and fire departments, and college students preparing for a career in health and fitness.

The YMCA faculty and exercise physiology consultants for the training courses have met on a regular basis to maintain a high standard of equality and consistency for all the courses held in different locations throughout the country. This group standardizes the procedures and creates a written exam and description of testing procedures. The five-day training course consists of the following required elements:

1. Fourteen hours of basic science review, which is taught by exercise physiology consultants with appropriate credentials. The review includes lectures on the anatomy and physiology of the muscular and cardiorespiratory systems, metabolic equations, biomechanics, and body composition.

2. Twelve hours of laboratory learning and practice, which provides trainees with hands-on experience in administering the test battery.

3. Ten hours of lecture on organization, administration, marketing, and the application of the training back at the local YMCA.

4. A practical test that requires each candidate to explain all the test items in the YMCA test battery to a participant, demonstrate when necessary, administer the test, record and score the results, and explain and interpret the results to the participant.

5. A standardized two-hour written test on all the lecture and laboratory material.

In 1989, after 11 years of training and certification experience, the Y added another requirement for certification. After each candidate returned to his or her respective YMCA or other facility, he or she had to administer the fitness test battery 10 times prior to certification. Throughout the past 10 years both faculty and students have said that this unique requirement has been invaluable in helping students learn to administer the tests correctly. No other fitness testing certification has this important requirement.

After completing the 10 test batteries, the candidate sends the data from the completed test batteries to the course faculty member, who checks the accuracy of the tests, tabulates the scores, and sends them to the YMCA of the USA to be added to a growing database. This database grows by approximately 3,000 scores each year, which are used to formulate the YMCA norm tables. These norms are incorporated into this book.

In the 1990s local YMCA programs grew in number and variety, and the increased number of YMCA of the USA training and certification courses available reflect that growth. In addition to the Fitness Specialist, certifications such as YMCA Personal Training Instructor, Healthy Back Instructor, and YMCA

Group Exercise Instructor are now offered. A description of the YMCA of the USA certification system and a listing of national certification courses in health and fitness are presented in chapter 2.

YMCA Fitness Assessment Protocol

The YMCA Fitness Assessment protocol, which mainly consists of the tests from the original Y's Way to Physical Fitness, is presented in chapter 6 of this book. One of the factors that makes the YMCA Fitness Testing and Assessment Program unique is that the same basic tests for cardiorespiratory endurance, body composition, flexibility, and muscular strength and endurance have been performed consistently by YMCAs across the country. This consistency has enabled the YMCA to collect results from individuals of all ages and abilities to create a norm database.

Through the years health and fitness directors have become familiar with and have been satisfied by the YMCA fitness assessment philosophy, test battery, and protocols. In this new book, we are not abandoning the principles established in Y's Way to Physical Fitness. The test battery initially presented in that book, which was created by dozens of experts representing all the specialties within sports medicine, has been used successfully and extensively for many years. Instead, this book is an update of the material with revisions and changes reflecting new information and research. It includes new norms, the best adult fitness norms available anywhere. We have noted certain problems, considerations, corrections, and adaptations discovered through years of using this test battery; these concerns are addressed in this text.

Purpose of This Book

When Y's Way to Physical Fitness was first being developed in the late 1960s, enough material was collected to write two or three volumes. The editors did not want, however, to write a book that covered everything from tests and measurements, the physiology of exercise, and the administration of physical education. Instead, they chose to write a straightforward manual that gave YMCA fitness directors information on how to organize and administer a fitness program and how to conduct a fitness testing program that could be understood and interpreted to participants. That text would contain all the necessary forms for each physical fitness test and give norms for each test item. They produced a concise, readable, well-formatted book that the staff could use. That philosophy is the basis of this book as well.

The primary purpose of this book is to present information on how to administer the YMCA Fitness Assessment protocol. We include the standard testing protocol, national norm tables for adults, and the rationale behind various tests. The material is pertinent to anyone administering fitness assessment programs. Chapters 3 and 4 also help readers to understand the basic exercise physiology behind the test battery, which in turn helps them to understand the tests and better interpret test results.

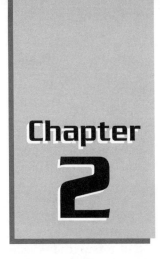

Chapter 2

YMCA Health and Fitness Programs

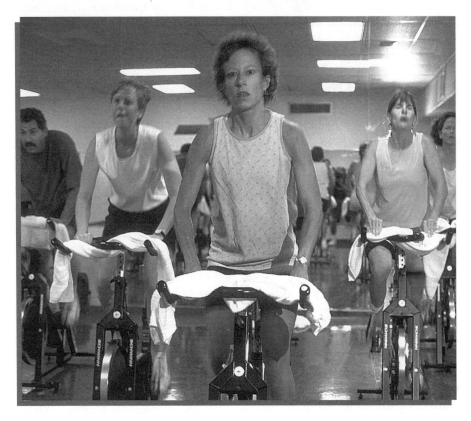

This chapter explains the YMCA mission, program objectives, health and fitness philosophy, and certifications available through the YMCA of the USA.

YMCA Mission, Objectives, and Philosophy

For more than 150 years the YMCA has perpetuated its mission through its programs, and health and fitness programs have been a key part of this effort.

YMCA Mission

The mission of the YMCA of the USA is to put Christian principles into practice through programs that build a healthy spirit, mind, and body for all.

YMCA Program Objectives

The goal of YMCA health and fitness programs, as in all YMCA programs, is to help people grow spiritually, mentally, and physically. To accomplish this goal, all YMCA programs address seven specific objectives, which are listed here. Subgoals or examples are listed under each category.

GROW PERSONALLY. Build self-esteem and self-reliance.

Develop self-esteem. People who are involved in YMCA programs gain a greater sense of their own worth. They learn to treat themselves and others with respect. High self-esteem helps people of all ages to build strong, healthy relationships and overcome obstacles in life so that they can reach their full potential.

DEVELOP CHARACTER. Develop moral and ethical behavior based on Christian principles.

Practice values. The YMCA has been helping people develop values for 150 years. Founded originally to bring men to God through Christ, the YMCA has evolved into an inclusive organization that helps people of all faiths develop values and behavior that are consistent with Judeo-Christian principles. The YMCA believes that the four values of honesty, respect, responsibility, and caring are essential for character development. Emphasis is on building a core set of values shared by the world's major religions and by people from all walks of life.

IMPROVE PERSONAL AND FAMILY RELATIONSHIPS. Learn to care, communicate, and cooperate with family and friends.

Support families. Today YMCAs are embracing families of all kinds and are more flexible in responding to their needs. Not only do Ys strengthen families through their own programs, but YMCA staff are increasingly being trained to help families in need or in crisis to find other community supports that can help. YMCAs plan programs and events with today's busy, sometimes frantic, families in mind. Families also get involved in helping plan and run Y family programs. The idea is to program with families, not just for them.

APPRECIATE DIVERSITY. Respect people of different ages, abilities, incomes, races, religions, cultures, and beliefs.

Reflect the diversity of the community. The United States population is diverse in terms of religion, race, ethnicity, age, income, abilities, and lifestyle. YMCAs must assess their membership to see whether it reflects the diversity of their communities. Diversity is a source of strength. The YMCA strives to foster an environment where everyone is treated with respect and is able to contribute to the larger community. Diversity should be celebrated, not merely tolerated.

BECOME BETTER LEADERS AND SUPPORTERS. Learn the give and take necessary to work toward the common good.

Promote leadership development through volunteerism. Volunteer leadership drives the YMCA, and today we place a renewed emphasis on providing meaningful volunteer opportunities for all kinds of people, especially youth and families. The Y encourages people to move from program participation to deeper levels of involvement, including volunteer leadership. Volunteer leadership will enrich their lives, their YMCAs, and their communities.

DEVELOP SPECIFIC SKILLS. Acquire new knowledge and ways to grow in spirit, mind, and body.

Build life skills. YMCA programs help people succeed in their daily lives through programs that build self-reliance, practical skills, and good values. Such programs include employment programs for teens and programs that support activities of daily living for seniors.

HAVE FUN. Enjoy life!

Fun and humor are essential qualities of all programs and contribute to people feeling good about themselves and the YMCA.

YMCA Health and Fitness Philosophy

The YMCA takes the wellness, or holistic, approach to health and fitness. Its programs are organized around the principle that the body, mind, and spirit make up a united whole. A strong component of this approach to health and fitness includes a focus on prevention.

One of the main goals shared by all YMCA programs is helping people to live a long and productive life and have fun living it. That's the way the YMCA approaches exercise. It's not something we do just for our bodies. Physical fitness is a way of life that requires education in good nutrition, proper exercise, avoidance of drug and alcohol abuse, coping with stress, and structuring life to lessen problems posed by chronic ailments such as arthritis, cancer, and heart disease.

Today, emphasis on prevention stretches from the field of medicine to the field of insurance. People understand how important their daily actions can be for long-term health. The YMCA is a major provider of affordable health and fitness programs, which encourage self-improvement. Our membership is culturally diverse, made up of people of all ages and abilities.

A variety of national training and certification programs in health and fitness are available to YMCA staff and volunteers. YMCA standards generally meet or exceed those required by local and state licensing boards. Since the 1880s the Y has been a leader in the field. Its own health and fitness professionals number in the thousands. The Y has also served as a training ground for recreation and physical education professionals outside the Y, for the health and fitness industry, and for corporate wellness programs.

It was in 1891 that a Y physical education leader created an enduring symbol for the YMCA, the now-familiar red triangle. To this day that triangle symbolizes the association's commitment to helping people build healthy lives, healthy families, and healthy communities.

Because exercise and physical education have been YMCA staples for so long, the Y already had health and fitness centers in all 50 states in the 1970s, when the pursuit of good health turned into a national passion. The YMCA is still a leader today, with state-of-the-art facilities, equipment, and exercise programs.

The YMCA believes that exercise and health education are important and should be provided for people of all ages and abilities. Most Ys look for ways in which all members of a family can participate in physical activity, which helps in developing positive family relationships.

The YMCA is a community service organization for all—a warm, relaxed place led by volunteers and run by well-trained and helpful employees who maintain its wholesome atmosphere. The YMCA encourages independence and self-reliance. This approach, combined with an open-door policy, has established YMCAs as true community centers, with programs and activities for everyone from the very fit to those with permanent disabilities, from the very young to older adults.

YMCA members and participants have a wide range of exercise alternatives from which to choose. Working out in the strength training center or keeping step in group exercise classes help many stay in shape. Others want more intensive exercise, perhaps to train for an upcoming event. And some want less intensity, perhaps just enough to help them build the strength and find the motivation to move from the couch to the walking path. Whatever the goal, a YMCA staff member will help the individual draw up a realistic plan to achieve it, offer encouragement along the way, and help map out a new direction when the goal is reached.

The YMCA strives to recognize the unique needs of individuals who join our organization. The mission of the YMCA comes alive for each person when we help that individual reach his or her unique potential through our programs and services. In helping people improve their health, we tailor the program to meet people's individual needs by doing the following:

- Assessing their current health status
- Discussing their personal goals
- Discussing their areas of interest
- Examining the roadblocks that are preventing them from achieving their goals
- Setting realistic short- and long-term goals based on their interests and activities
- Getting them involved in programs designed to meet their personal goals

YMCA Health and Fitness Leadership Training and Certification

The primary factor in conducting successful health and fitness programs is the strength of the leadership. The YMCA has traditionally been a respected leader in health and fitness programs, due largely to having instructors qualified by experience, knowledge, training, and up-to-date information.

The leadership training and certification program for YMCA health and fitness programs has developed throughout the 150-year history of the organization and evolved to keep pace with this dynamic field. The Y's approach to the training program is to teach specific skills, leadership qualities, and technical information to prepare participants to teach courses. The trainings are not, however, intended to provide complete preparation for local YMCA instructors. It is incumbent upon YMCA staff to supplement instructors' training with on-the-job and other educational experiences, including guidance from supervisors, technical workshops and seminars, and networking with other instructors.

Let's now look at the levels of leadership certification available and the training events that lead to certification.

Levels of Leadership Certifications

Five levels of leadership certification are available through the YMCA: Basic, Instructor, Director, Trainer, and Faculty.

1. *Basic:* The Basic level is for individuals interested in assisting an instructor in a health and fitness class. Staff certified at this level receive training by working with YMCA instructors, training at their local YMCA, and attending YMCA certification courses. Following are Basic-level courses:

- Principles of YMCA Health and Fitness
- Continuing Education Courses for YMCA Group Exercise and Personal Training Instructors

2. *Instructor:* The YMCA Health and Fitness Instructor level is for people providing primary leadership to YMCA programs. To become certified as an Instructor, an individual must meet all prerequisites for and complete a YMCA of the USA certification course. Here is a listing of Instructor-level courses:

- YMCA Group Exercise Instructor
- YMCA Personal Training Instructor
- Healthy Back Instructor
- Prenatal Exercise Instructor
- Youth Fitness Instructor
- YMCA Walk Reebok Instructor
- YMCA Walk Reebok Distance/Interval Instructor
- Active Older Adult Exercise Instructor (land)
- YMCA/IDEA Get Real Weight Management Instructor
- YMCA Martial Arts Exercise Instructor

3. *Director:* This level certifies participants to administer programs and to train staff members and volunteers at their own YMCA. These are the two Director-level courses:

- Fitness Specialist
- YMCA Personal Fitness Program Director

4. *Trainer:* This level is for individuals interested in training and certifying other YMCA Instructors by leading YMCA of the USA Instructor courses. These individuals must meet all requirements of Trainer courses and be approved by the YMCA of the USA. Trainer courses are offered in all of the programs listed for the Instructor and Director levels.

5. *Faculty:* The top YMCA trainers in the United States are certified as faculty members, qualifying them to teach the Trainer courses. The Faculty level is offered only at the invitation of the YMCA of the USA. Faculty members are trained and certified at a Program Training Academy conducted by the YMCA of the USA.

Certification Training Events

All YMCA of the USA program certification training is delivered by YMCA staff members across the country who are certified as trainers or faculty and volunteer their time to conduct the training workshops. The YMCA of the USA Membership and Program Development Group is responsible for overseeing the entire national training network. YMCA certification courses are offered in two different ways:

1. *Local Cluster Training Events:* Sanctioned by the YMCA of the USA Field Program Coordinator and conducted by certified trainers, these training courses can be hosted by any local YMCA.

2. *National Program Schools:* The YMCA of the USA sanctions over 20 Program Schools annually in various cities around the country, with a number of different certification trainings available. A list of Program Schools is available from the YMCA of the USA.

At the conclusion of all certification events, the trainer completes the certification form, listing all participants who have successfully completed all of the training requirements. The form and certification fee of $8.00 per person is sent to the YMCA of the USA national office in Chicago for processing, and certification cards are sent to everyone who completes the course successfully.

Contacts for More Information on YMCA of the USA Programs

For YMCA of the USA certification information:
YMCA of the USA
Membership and Program Development Group
101 North Wacker Dr.
Chicago, IL 60606
800-USA-YMCA

For YMCA program resource materials:
YMCA Program Store
P.O. Box 5076
Champaign, IL 61825
800-747-0089

For information on YMCA trainings in your area, contact your YMCA of the USA Field Office:

YMCA of the USA
East Field Office
661 Moore Rd.
King of Prussia, PA 19406
610-337-3116
800-962-2336

YMCA of the USA
Mid-America Field Office
800 LaSalle Ave.
Minneapolis, MN 55402
612-332-1548
800-248-9622

YMCA of the USA
South Field Office
100 Edgewood Ave. NE
Atlanta, GA 30303
404-521-0352
800-359-9622

YMCA of the USA
West Field Office
1650 South Amphlett Blvd.
San Mateo, CA 94402
415-574-2003
800-877-9622

Part II

Basics
of
Anatomy,
Physiology,
and
Kinesiology

Chapter 3

Skeletal Muscles

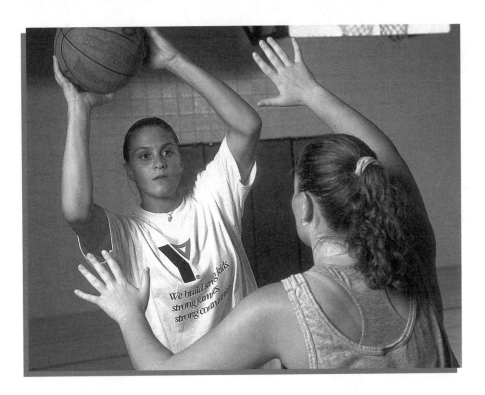

Many excellent exercise physiology and biology textbooks are available for in-depth reading on muscle anatomy, physiology, and kinesiology. Rather than try to replace those, we want to present to you some basic anatomical and physiological facts and concepts about muscles that will help you understand how the muscle is structured, how it works, and how it changes under the stress of exercise. The concepts presented here are basic and simplified, but it is our hope that after reading this chapter you will continue your study with more advanced references (some of which can be found in the reading list at the end of this chapter).

In this chapter we start by discussing the three classifications of muscles and their actions. We then turn to teaching the names of muscles and joint movements, followed by a description of some of the properties of muscle tissue and the possible types of muscle contraction. We end the chapter with information on muscle fibers and how they are affected by strength training.

Classification of Muscles

All physical activity involves muscles because it is the muscles' action on bones that allows us to move. If asked to name a muscle, we might name the biceps, triceps, or quads. All of these are *locomotor* muscles, or muscles that allow us to move. Other types of muscles can be found in the body, however. Muscles fall into three classifications determined by their location in the body, their microscopic appearance, or how they are controlled by the nervous system.

Classification by Location

The early anatomists were called *gross anatomists*; they examined the body as they saw it with the naked eye. They worked on cadavers. When they named muscles, they did so according to where the muscles were located in the body. If a muscle was attached to a bone, or the skeleton, for example, it was called a *skeletal* muscle. The skeletal muscles and bones make up a lever system within the body that permits movement.

Other muscles in the body are not attached to bones. These include the muscles in the walls of the stomach and intestines, the muscles in the walls of arteries and veins that allow the blood vessels to constrict and dilate, and the muscles that control entrances or exits to hollow organs like the stomach (sphincter muscles). (By the way, sit-ups exercise not the stomach muscles but rather the abdominal muscles, which are skeletal muscles. The stomach muscles are used during digestion.) Nonlocomotor muscles are found wherever there are blood vessels; these muscles were observed by the early anatomists mostly in the abdominal cavity (the viscera) and were therefore called *visceral* muscles.

Yet another muscle exists that is so unique it forms a class all by itself. This is the heart or *cardiac* muscle.

Thus, the three kinds of muscles in the body as identified by location are skeletal, visceral, and cardiac. All muscles can be put into one of these three subdivisions.

Classification by Microscopic Appearance

With the advent of the microscope, anatomists started studying the human body at a cellular level. Scientists who studied muscles with a microscope were called *histologists*. When histologists observed muscle cells through the microscope, they wanted to create a classification that was based on muscles' microscopic appearance, so a second system of classifying muscles was added.

Histologists observed that skeletal muscle cells had light and dark bands along the length of the tubelike cell, so they called these *striated* muscles. The visceral muscle cells did not have these light and dark bands, so these muscles were called *nonstriated,* or *smooth,* muscles.

Histologically, the heart muscle once again was unique. Its cells had striations, but they were not regular like those in the skeletal muscle. Instead the striations were interconnected with each other in a latticelike pattern, and so the heart muscle has sometimes been called a *branch-striated,* or *syncytium*, muscle.

This second method of classifying the muscles by their microscopic appearance again places all the body's muscles into one of three subdivisions: striated, smooth, or syncytium.

Classification by Nervous System Control

Neurologists studied anatomy from a different perspective. These physiologists were interested in how the body controls functions through the nervous system, so they classified muscles according to how the muscles were innervated.

Some muscles can be innervated (contracted) at will (volitionally) and are controlled by the central nervous system. Neurologists named these muscles *voluntary* muscles. Other muscles, like those in the walls of the stomach and intestines, cannot be controlled voluntarily, as they are under control of the autonomic nervous system. The same applies to the cardiac muscle. These muscles were called *involuntary* muscles. A few muscles, such as the muscles of respiration, can be controlled voluntarily but also contract automatically. These were called *voluntary/involuntary* muscles.

This third method of classifying muscles was developed based on how the muscles were controlled by the nervous system. It groups them according to whether they are voluntary, involuntary, or voluntary/involuntary.

Three Classifications

Table 3.1 presents the three methods of classifying muscles and the three subdivisions of muscle types under each method.

Table 3.1 Classification of Muscles

Location	Microscopic appearance	Nervous system control
Skeletal	Striated	Voluntary
Visceral	Smooth or nonstriated	Involuntary
Cardiac	Syncytium or branch-striated	Voluntary/involuntary

Although only three kinds of muscles exist in the body, each muscle can be named using one of the three classifications. For example, the biceps can be classified as a skeletal muscle, a striated muscle, or a voluntary muscle. In most physical activity, we are primarily interested in skeletal muscles.

Muscle Concepts

To understand how muscles work during exercise and which muscles are used, we need to review some basic anatomical and physiological concepts about locomotor muscles. This review addresses muscle action (how muscles move), muscle antagonists, action around a joint, and two-joint action.

Muscle Action

A skeletal muscle acts like a rubber band that has been stretched and is trying to return to its normal length. It either pulls or tries to shorten. If you nailed a strong piece of rubber tubing to a gate and then stretched it across the hinge and nailed it to the adjacent fence, the stretched rubber band would try to shorten and open the gate (see figure 3.1). The fence would not move because it's immovable; the gate would open, however, because the hinge is movable. The action of the biceps, which crosses the arm over the hinge of the elbow, is the same as the rubber band example just described (see figure 3.2).

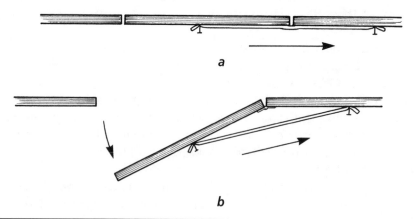

a

b

Figure 3.1 Rubber tubing (a) nailed to a gate and stretched across the hinge to the adjacent fence (b) tries to shorten and open the gate.

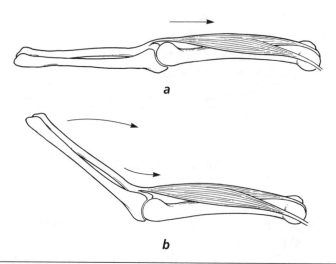

a

b

Figure 3.2 The biceps crosses the elbow to create movement in the joint.

This example illustrates two important concepts. First, just as the rubber band must cross the hinge to create the movement, the muscle also must cross a joint to create movement around that joint. Second, when the gate is closed, the rubber band is parallel to the fence and gate (see figure 3.3). The rubber band exerts little pull on the gate because it is pulling along the line of the fence into the hinge. But once the gate starts to open, the rubber bands pulls at an angle and can operate strongly (see figure 3.4). The pull of the rubber band is strongest when the gate is open at 90°.

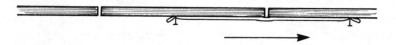

Figure 3.3 The closed gate.

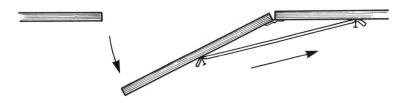

Figure 3.4   The rubber band pulls as the gate starts to open.

The pull of the rubber band on the gate is similar to the biceps example. When the elbow is straight, the pull of the biceps is parallel to the bone and does not have a strong action (see figure 3.5). As the elbow starts to bend, however, its action on the lower arm becomes strong because the angle of pull is improved (see figure 3.6). The mechanical efficiency is greatest when the attachment of the biceps is at a 90° angle to the bones. Variable resistance machines for weight training were designed with the angle of attachment in mind; different amounts of resistance are needed at different angles of a joint, as the force exerted by the muscle changes with varying angles.

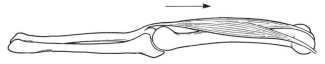

Figure 3.5   When the elbow is straight, the biceps does not have a strong action.

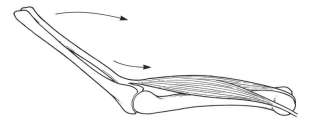

Figure 3.6   As the elbow starts to bend, the angle of pull is improved.

Antagonist Muscles

Skeletal muscles are arranged in antagonistic, opposite pairs. In our example of the gate, the rubber band attached to the top of the fence will open the gate, but if we want the gate to close, the rubber band is useless. The rubber band cannot push the gate closed; it can only pull. If we were to attach another rubber band to the bottom of the gate and hinge, the bottom band could rebound from a stretched position when the gate is opened and then shorten to pull the gate closed (see figure 3.7).

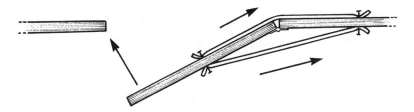

Figure 3.7   A second rubber strip attached to the gate will rebound and shorten, pulling the gate closed.

At this point our rubber band example falters, as we have to take the tension off the first rubber band for the second one to work. We cannot do this with rubber tubing, however, unless we disconnect it. But in the human body, the removal of tension from one half of an antagonistic pair of muscles can be done through the nervous system. The biceps on the front of the upper arm, for example, is innervated (a nerve impulse causes the muscle to contract) and shortened, which causes the elbow to bend. The triceps on the back of the upper arm relaxes and stretches as the elbow bends. To straighten the elbow, the reverse occurs; the biceps relaxes and the triceps shortens, creating the opposite movement (see figure 3.8).

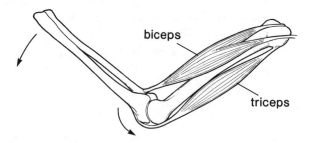

Figure 3.8 The biceps and triceps work together to create antagonist action.

All our joints are surrounded by muscles arranged in this antagonist manner, with one muscle performing one action and the opposite muscle performing the opposite action. Picture in your mind the muscles acting like puppets on a string: one string makes one movement, the other string the opposite movement.

Note that because we live in an environment with gravity, the antagonist occasionally is gravity itself. Standing and raising the arms sideways, for example, is a result of the shoulder abductors crossing the shoulder joint (see figure 3.9). Antagonist muscles exist—the adductors—to take the arms back to the side, but because gravity lowers the arms to the sides, the adductors (or antagonists) are

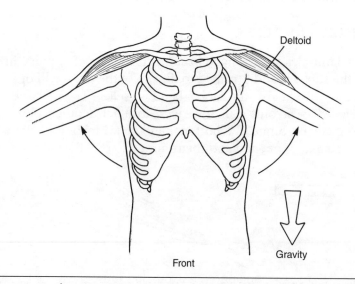

Figure 3.9 Gravity acts as the antagonist in some situations.

not needed. The effect of gravity on the arms would be different if you were standing in water. If you stood neck deep in a swimming pool you would be almost weightless (see figure 3.10). To raise your arms to the sides, you would again use the shoulder abductors, but to return them to the sides you would have to contract the adductors because gravity would not exert enough pull to lower them down.

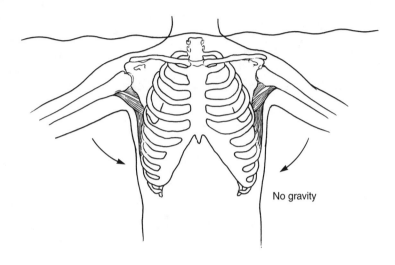

No gravity

Figure 3.10   In water, the body is almost weightless, and gravity has no effect against the water's buoyancy.

Muscle Action Around a Joint

A muscle must cross a joint to cause the joint to move. A good example is the abdominal muscles. The abdominal muscles arise (or originate) on the pelvic bone (hips) and insert on the rib cage. They pull the front of the chest down to the hips (spine or trunk flexion), curving the spine forward. They do not cross the hip joint, so they cannot move the body to a sitting or a jackknife position (hip flexion). The muscles that cause the hips to move to a full sitting position are the hip flexors, not the abdominals (see figure 3.11).

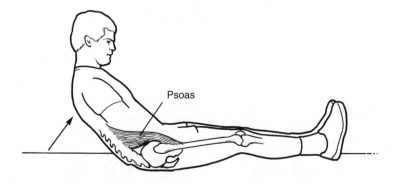

Psoas

Figure 3.11   The hip flexors, not the abdominal muscles, cause the body to move to a full sitting position.

In a full sit-up (see figure 3.12), the abdominals work to curl the spine forward (rolling up). When their action is complete (at approximately 30°), they hold the curled position and the hip flexors take over to "bend" the hips into a complete sit-up position. The hip flexors *do* cross the hip joint, originating on the lumbar vertebra and inserting on the upper femur. As gravity works to return the body to the prone position, the hip flexors and then the abdominals again allow the body to return to the starting or lying position (eccentric contraction of the hip flexors and spine flexors). A full sit-up uses both the abdominals (curling up) and the hip flexors (jackknifing at the hips). When the person returns to the starting position, the same muscles contract eccentrically. Full sit-ups are no longer as prevalent in exercise routines because the half sit-up is enough to work the abdominals completely. In addition, engaging the hip flexors can cause strain on the low back.

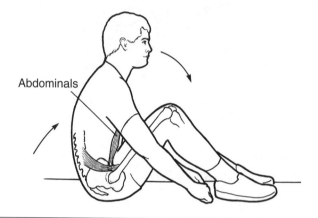

Abdominals

Figure 3.12   In a full sit-up, both the abdominal muscles and the hip flexors are used.

Two-Joint Action

If a muscle crosses two joints, it will operate both joints and be responsible for two movements. If it crosses three joints, it will bring about three movements. Let's look again at the biceps example discussed previously (see figure 3.13). The biceps crosses the elbow joint and the shoulder joint. The biceps originates on the front of the scapula just under the clavicle and inserts on the radius (lower arm), so the biceps is crossing the front of the shoulder joint and the front of the elbow joint. We already know that the biceps flexes the elbow. Because the biceps also crosses the front of the shoulder joint, it pulls the whole arm upward (shoulder flexion), so the biceps is said to be both a flexor of the elbow and a flexor of the arm or shoulder.

Because the biceps attaches to the radius, it has yet another action (see figure 3.14). The radius and ulna lie together. The ulna joins the humerus to form the elbow joint, which flexes and extends. The radius is not part of this joint but instead lies to the outside and is responsible for pronation and supination, which allow the lower arm and hand to rotate longitudinally. In pronation the radius and ulna cross each other, causing the palm to face the back; in supination the radius and ulna lie parallel to each other, causing the palm to face front.

To illustrate the difference between elbow flexion and extension and pronation and supination, try the following exercise. To demonstrate flexion and extension of the elbow joint, place the hand palm up (supinated) on a table with

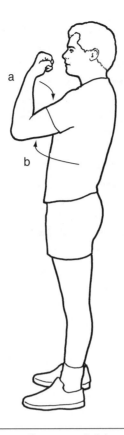

Figure 3.13 The biceps acts as (a) elbow flexor and (b) arm or shoulder flexor.

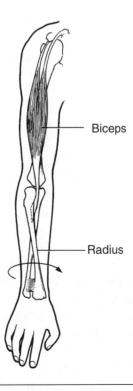

Biceps

Radius

Figure 3.14 The radius and ulna cross each other during pronation.

the elbow slightly flexed. Keeping the hand supinated, flex the elbow and move the palm toward the shoulder (flexion) and then return the hand to the table (extension). Now, leave the hand (palm up) on the table, again keeping the elbow slightly flexed; roll the hand over so that the palm is now facing the table (pronation). Rotate the hand back to the palm-up position (supination). Pronation and supination of the hand (or more correctly the radial-ulna joint) is a lower arm movement only.

The biceps muscle inserts on the upper inside of the radius. When the hand is supinated (starting position), the biceps insertion is anterior (toward the front) and medial (closest to the body) on the radius (between the radius and ulna); but when the hand is pronated, the biceps attachment goes between the radius and ulna so that it is posterior. (The radius rotates longitudinally on its axis in pronation and supination, as in figure 3.14.) When the biceps contracts, it pulls its attachment on the radius forward, causing supination. Because the biceps crosses three joints (shoulder, elbow, and radial-ulna) it acts on all three, resulting in three actions: supination (radial-ulna joint), elbow flexion (elbow joint), and arm or shoulder flexion (shoulder joint).

Joint Movements

Most strength training books contain muscle charts naming all the skeletal muscles, such as the biceps, triceps, latissimus dorsi, pectoralis, and quadriceps. Learning the names for all the muscles, however, requires a lot of memorization, and the muscle names may be quickly forgotten if they are not repeated frequently. An easier and more useful way to identify muscles is to learn the movements for each joint, which you probably can do in 15 to 30 minutes, and then refer to muscles by the joint action they can create. For example, the muscles that cause the elbow to flex are called the elbow flexors. Joint and muscle movements are listed next. Remember that these basic movements start from the anatomical starting position, which is feet together facing forward with the hands supinated (palms facing forward with the arms by the sides). This position is shown in figure 3.15.

To illustrate the importance of the starting position, stand erect with your hands at your sides in a normal standing position. In this position, the palms of your hands are facing your thighs (pronated). Now bend or flex your elbows. Your elbows go sideways, and the shoulder joints also move. The resulting position is the "arms akimbo" (hands on the hips) position. By contrast, stand in the anatomical position with your palms forward (hands supinated) and again bend or flex your elbows. This is a completely different movement: the elbows bend and the forearms and hands move forward and up. The shoulder joint does not move. Elbow flexion from the anatomical starting position is true elbow flexion; elbow flexion from a normal standing position, however, is not a true anatomical joint movement. All anatomy textbook muscular actions are described as originating from the anatomical starting position.

In the following sections, each joint movement is named and explained, and the joint that makes that movement is listed. To learn the movements, practice each one, always beginning from the anatomical starting position.

Note that the movements described next are not named uniformly. A movement occurs around a joint, and the movement can be named for the joint or for the body segment below the joint. Which of these names is chosen is up to the user or is determined by common usage. For example, one can describe shoul-

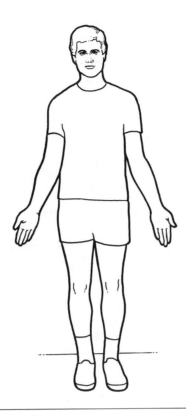

Figure 3.15 Anatomical starting position.

der flexion (the shoulder being the joint) or arm flexion (the arm being the body segment below the joint), elbow flexion or forearm flexion, hip flexion or leg flexion, and so on.

Because one action of a joint is followed by the opposite action, which returns the joint to its starting anatomical position, joint movements are usually presented in pairs, such as flexion and extension. If the joint can move beyond its starting position, it also may have another term to explain that added movement. Hyperextension, for example, occurs when a joint moves beyond the starting position.

Note that the terms listed here (except for a few) must be followed or preceded by a joint or limb name; they cannot stand alone. Thus you would not refer simply to *flexion* but instead to *elbow flexion, flexion of the elbow,* or *forearm flexion.*

Let's now look at the joint movements, which include flexion, extension, and hyperextension; abduction and adduction; rotation; and a few other actions and movements.

Flexion, Extension, Hyperextension

Flexion usually means that the angle of the joint is decreasing, whereas extension usually means that the angle is increasing. Some exceptions exist. The following are the 10 joints that flex and extend and, in some cases, hyperextend (for the ankle, plantar and dorsiflex). Now stand, assume the anatomical position, and try the following movements. Remember to always start at and return to the anatomical position. Practice each of these movements 5 to 10 times, naming them as you perform them. Remember to include a joint or limb name with each action, such as flexion of the elbow or hip flexion.

	Flexion	Extension	Hyperextension
Fingers (figure A)	Curl up the fingers.	Straighten the fingers.	Curve the fingers back beyond the starting position.
Wrist or hand (figure B)	Move the hand forward and up with the fingers straight.	Return the fingers to the anatomical position.	Bend the straight hand backward.
Elbow or forearm (figure C)	Bend the elbow.	Straighten the elbow.	None (normally)
Shoulder or arm (figure D)	Bring the straight arm forward and up.	Return the straight arm to the anatomical position.	Move the straight arm backward beyond the starting position.

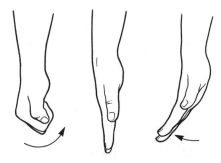

Figure A Finger flexion, extension, and hyperextension.

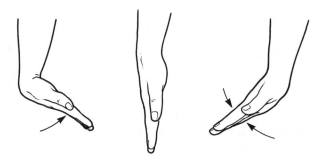

Figure B Wrist flexion, extension, and hyperextension.

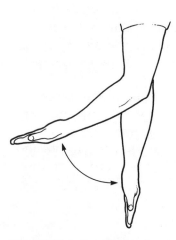

Figure C Elbow flexion and extension.

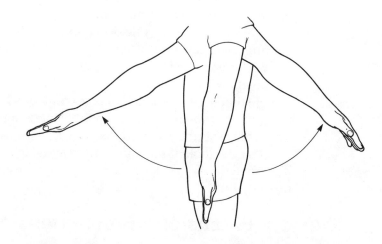

Figure D Shoulder or arm flexion, extension, and hyperextension.

	Flexion	Extension	Hyperextension
Neck or head (figure E)	Drop the head forward onto the chest.	Return the head to the anatomical position.	Move the head backward beyond the starting anatomical position.
Spine or trunk (figure F)	Curve the spine forward. Do not bend at the hips.	Straighten the spine, returning to the anatomical position.	Curve the spine backward beyond the anatomical position.
Hip or leg* (figure G)	Keep the spine straight and bend at the hips.	Return to the starting anatomical position.	Lean backward beyond the starting anatomical position.

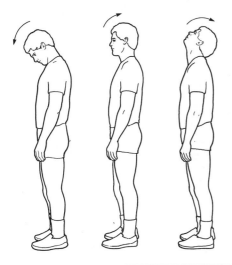

Figure E Head or neck flexion, extension, and hyperextension.

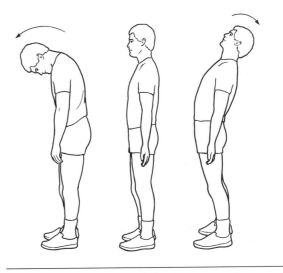

Figure F Spine or trunk flexion, extension, and hyperextension.

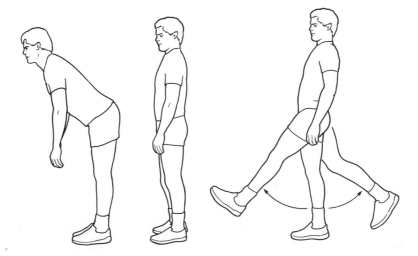

Figure G Hip or leg flexion, extension, and hyperextension.

*This same action could also be done by raising the leg forward (leg or hip flexion), then returning it to the starting position (leg or hip extension) or taking it beyond the starting position (hip or leg hyperextension).

	Flexion	Extension	Hyperextension
Knee or lower leg (figure H)	Bend the knee.	Straighten the knee.	None (normally)
Ankle or foot** (figure I)	Point the foot or rise up on the toes (plantar flexion).	Return to the starting anatomical position (dorsiflexion).	None
Toes (figure J)	Curl the toes under the foot.	Return the toes to the starting position.	Raise the toes from the starting position.

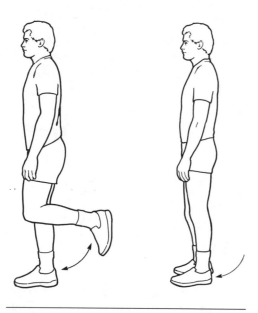

Figure H   Knee flexion and extension.

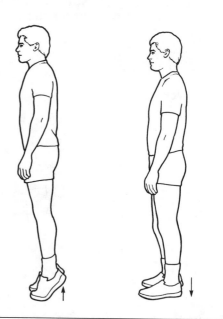

Figure I   Plantar and dorsal flexion.

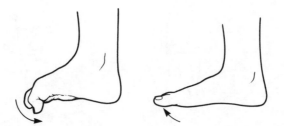

Figure J   Toe flexion and extension.

** The ankle or foot is a special case. The terms *flexion* and *extension* can be used, in which case pointing the foot (or, if standing, rising up on the toes) is called *extension of the ankle* and returning to the starting position or elevating the foot is called *flexion of the ankle.* The two actions have also been referred to as *depression* and *elevation* of the foot. The preferable terms, however, when referring to the foot or ankle are *plantar flexion* and *dorsiflexion.*

Abduction and Adduction

Abduction is taking a body segment (limb) away from the centerline of the body (*ab* means "away from"). Adduction is moving the body segment (limb) toward the centerline of the body.

The following five joints abduct and adduct. Again, stand in the anatomical position and try the following movements. Practice each movement 5 to 10 times, naming the movement as you perform it. Again, remember to include a name before or after the movement, such as arm abduction or abduction of the arm.

	Abduction	Adduction
Fingers (figure K)	Keeping the thumb next to the hand, spread the fingers apart.	Return to the anatomical position.
Thumb (figure L)	Keeping the fingers together, move the thumb away from the hand.	Return to the anatomical position.
Arms or shoulders (figure M)	Move the arms sideways, away from the body.	Return the arms to the anatomical position.

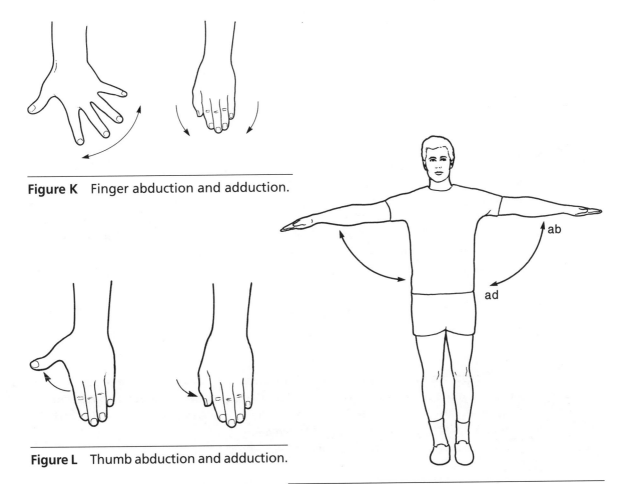

Figure K   Finger abduction and adduction.

Figure L   Thumb abduction and adduction.

Figure M   Arm or shoulder abduction and adduction.

	Abduction	Adduction
Legs or hips (figure N)	Move the legs apart or move one leg away from the centerline of the body (legs astride).	Return the leg(s) to the anatomical position.
Toes (figure O)	If you can, spread your toes apart.	Return the toes to the anatomical position.

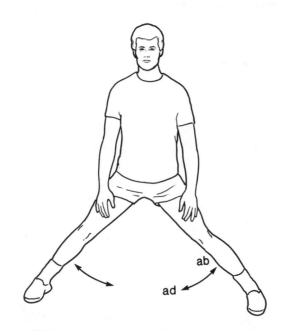

Figure N Leg or hip abduction and adduction.

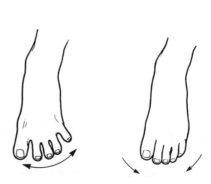

Figure O Toe abduction and adduction.

Rotation

Rotation of body parts is unique in that some parts rotate toward and away from the centerline of the body, such as the arms and the legs, whereas others only rotate to the left or to the right, such as the head, neck, and trunk. Although the terms *inward* and *outward* are commonly used, the terms *medial* and *lateral* or *internal* and *external* may be substituted. Inward rotation, medial rotation, and internal rotation are all the same movement. Likewise, outward rotation, lateral rotation, and external rotation are the same.

INWARD ROTATION = Medial rotation = Internal rotation

OUTWARD ROTATION = Lateral rotation = External rotation

As mentioned previously, the lower arm (forearm) can also pronate or supinate. These are unique rotations and are restricted to the forearms (radial-ulna joint) only; the upper arm does not rotate during pronation and supination.

Another unique rotation is that of the foot. It rotates along its axis, and the movements are called *eversion* and *inversion*.

Try practicing the following rotation movements.

Rotations (to the left or to the right)		
Head or neck	Rotate the head to the left, return it to the anatomical position, and then rotate the head to the right.	
Trunk or spine	Rotate the trunk to the left, then return the trunk to the anatomical position; repeat to the right.	
	Inward rotation	**Outward rotation**
Shoulder or arm	Rotate the upper arm toward the body.	Return the arm to the anatomical position or beyond.
Hip or leg	Rotate the leg toward the centerline of the body.	Return the leg to the anatomical position or beyond.
	Pronation*	**Supination***
Forearm (or radial-ulna joint)	Keeping the upper arm stationary, rotate the palm of the hand from the forward anatomical position toward the body, facing backward.	Return the hand to the anatomical position, which is the supinated position.

*Because pronation and supination are unique to the hand (radial-ulna joint), these two movements do not need to be preceded or followed by a joint or limb name.

Eversion and Inversion

Eversion is sometimes called *pronation of the foot,* and inversion is sometimes called *supination of the foot.***

	Eversion	**Inversion**
Foot	Stand in the starting position and roll the foot onto the inside border of the foot.	Stand in the starting position and roll the foot onto the outside border of the foot.

**When the terms *pronation* or *supination* are used for foot movements, they must be followed by the word *foot,* as in *pronation of the foot.*

Lateral Flexion

Lateral flexion does not fit into any classification. It is not a true flexion. Only two body segments flex laterally, the head (neck) and the trunk (spine), and they move either to the left or right. Try these lateral movements:

■ *Lateral flexion of the head* (figure P): Starting in the anatomical position, move the head to the left while continuing to look forward, moving the left ear down to the shoulder. The return to the anatomical position has no name. The movement is lateral flexion, which can be performed to the left or to the right.

■ *Lateral flexion of the trunk (spine)* (figure Q): Starting in the anatomical position, bend the spine to the left while continuing to face forward so that the left hand slides down the left leg; this is lateral flexion of the trunk to the left. The return to the anatomical position has no name. Lateral flexion of the spine to the right is the opposite movement.

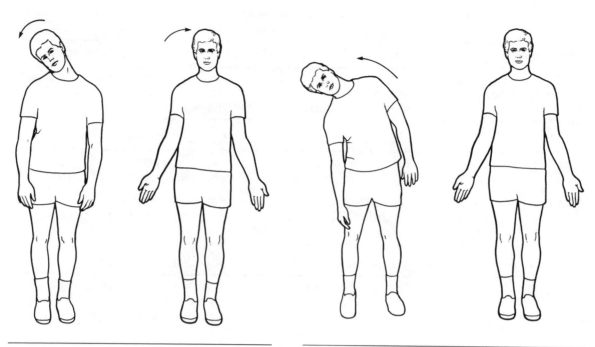

Figure P   Head or neck lateral flexion.   **Figure Q**   Spine or trunk lateral flexion.

Scapula Movements

The scapula (shoulder blade) has no bony attachment to the back of the skeleton. The scapula, arm, and clavicle make up the shoulder girdle. The shoulder girdle's only attachment to the skeleton is where the collarbone (clavicle) attaches to the sternum. The scapula has numerous muscles that attach to it, and it moves freely over the back. Muscles operate the movement of the scapula, and these movements are important to arm movement. Here are the six movements of the scapula:

- Elevation (raise)
- Depression (lower)
- Abduction (or protraction)
- Adduction (or retraction)
- Inward rotation
- Outward rotation

Practice these movements:

■ *Elevation and depression of the scapula* (figure R): Shrug the shoulders or lift the shoulders toward the ears (elevation). Return the shoulders to the normal, anatomical starting position (depression).

■ *Abduction and adduction of the scapula* (figure S): Round the shoulders to abduct the scapula, moving the scapula away from the spinal column (abduction). Now move the shoulders backward so the scapula moves toward the spinal column and the shoulders move closer together in the back (adduction).

■ *Inward and outward rotation of the scapula* (figure T): The scapula is free to rotate on the back. Think of it as an irregular wheel with the axle in the center. The reference point of this wheel is the inferior angle, and when the inferior angle moves toward the spinal column, it is called inward rotation of the scapula. When the inferior angle moves away from the spine, it is outward rotation of the scapula. Start from the anatomical position and raise a straight arm sideways and upward (arm abduction) for outward rotation of the scapula. Return to the anatomical position for inward rotation.

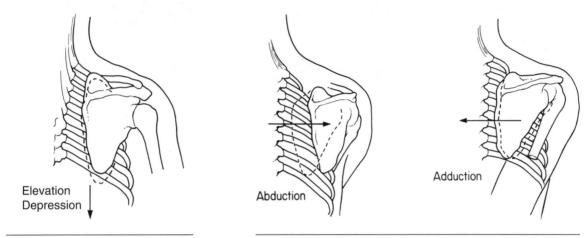

Figure R Scapula elevation and depression.

Figure S Scapula abduction and adduction.

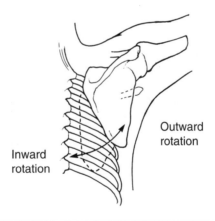

Figure T Scapula inward and outward rotation.

Self-Quiz

The following figure shows a series of actions. For each numbered figure, write the muscles involved in the joint movement in the corresponding numbered space. The answers are at the end of the chapter. Try to do this without looking at the answers.

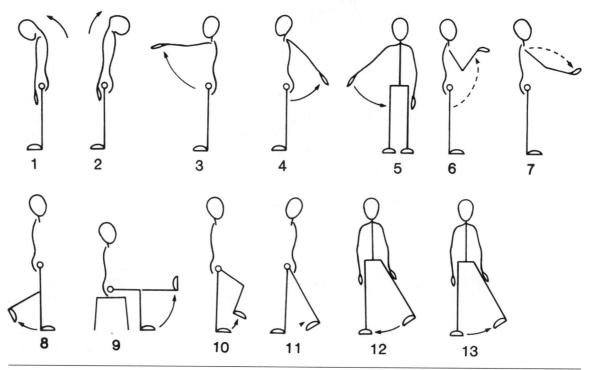

Muscle actions.

1. _____

2. _____

3. _____

4. _____

5. _____

6. _____

7. _____

8. _____

9. _____

10. _____

11. _____

12. _____

13. _____

Naming Muscle Groups by Muscle Actions

Now that you've learned the joint movements, you've also learned all the muscle actions, and you can use these actions to name various muscle groups. You can now refer to the elbow flexors, shoulder adductors, or knee extensors. To illustrate how to apply your knowledge of joint movements and muscle actions, let's look at a muscular analysis of the curl. The starting position is the anatomical position except that, to hold on to the barbell, the fingers are flexed using the finger flexor muscles. The primary movers during the curl are the elbow flexors. The curl, therefore, exercises or develops the elbow flexors. The list starting on page 44 shows the individual muscles that make up the elbow flexor group. The elbow flexors comprise all the muscles that are working in a curl. Too often it is said that curls develop the biceps, ignoring the fact that the biceps is just one of six elbow flexors. In fact, during the curl the brachialis is more of a true elbow flexor than the biceps. The muscles that cross the joint and cause the movement are indeed the muscles doing the work. Arm flexion is caused by the arm flexors, knee extension is done by the knee extensors, and so on.

Before you use this system, we need to define three other terms: prime movers, stabilizers, and neutralizers.

Prime Movers

Prime movers are muscles that do the major work to create a particular movement. In curls, for example, the prime movers are the elbow flexors; they do the main movement. In chin-ups, the prime movers are the elbow flexors and the shoulder extensors. The elbow flexors bend the elbows, and the shoulder extensors bring the elbows down to the sides (figure 3.16). Any muscle group, depending on the movement, can be a prime mover, and the prime movers change from exercise to exercise.

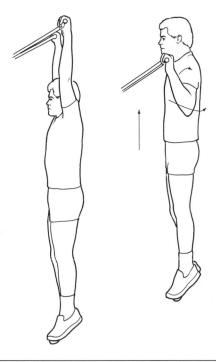

Figure 3.16 Prime movers in chin-up—elbow flexors and shoulder extensors.

Stabilizers

Stabilizers hold a body part in position during a movement. In push-ups the prime movers are the elbow extensors (which straighten the elbow) and the shoulder flexors (which bring the upper arm into the push-up position). If the rest of the body's muscles are relaxed during a push-up, however, the middle of the body would sag (see figure 3.17), which is extreme hyperextension of the spine and hips.

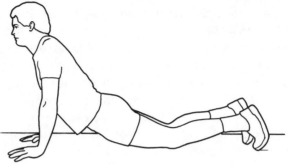

Figure 3.17 Push-up using only the prime movers.

The illustration in figure 3.18 shows the correct execution of a push-up. To keep the body in this position, resisting gravity, the person must contract the spine flexors and hip flexors. They cannot be contracted too much or the body position will change to a jackknife position. They must be contracted just enough to prevent the trunk from sagging and keep the body rigid. Muscles that stabilize the body are called *stabilizers*. In push-ups, the stabilizers are the spine flexors, hip flexors, knee extensors (to stop the knee from bending), and plantar flexors (pushing off the tendency of the body to move back).

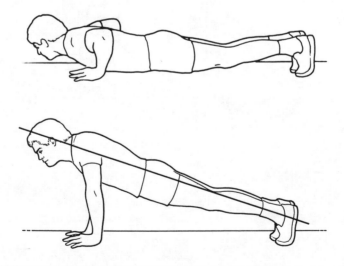

Figure 3.18 Push-up using the prime movers and the stabilizers holding the body straight.

Neutralizers

Although the term *neutralizers* will not be used often in this book, it is important to understand the concept. A neutralizer is a muscle that, when contracted, prevents (or neutralizes) an action of another muscle. For example, the biceps crosses three joints—the shoulder, the elbow, and the radial-ulna joint. The biceps acts on these three joints as follows:

- Shoulder joint (shoulder flexion)
- Elbow joint (elbow flexion)
- Radial-ulna joint (supination)

If we were to analyze the action involved in using a screwdriver to drive a screw into a piece of wood, we would find that the main movement involved is supination, so the biceps would be involved. The biceps also flexes the elbow, however, which, in this movement, is undesirable. Therefore, the triceps, which is an elbow extensor, is innervated to prevent (or neutralize) the flexion action of the biceps. In this situation, the triceps acts as a neutralizer. Imagine you are watching someone driving a screw into hard wood. The triceps contracts powerfully, but it does not help the movement; it is working to prevent the biceps from flexing the elbow. The biceps also tries to flex the shoulder. Because shoulder flexion is not needed in this movement, the shoulder extensors also are contracted to neutralize the shoulder flexion action of the biceps. As a result, only supination of the hand occurs.

Properties of Muscle Tissue

Muscle cells (or muscle tissue) have four characteristics that set them apart from other cells: contractility, extensibility, elasticity, and tonicity. Here are descriptions of each characteristic:

- *Contractility*—Contractility, or the ability to contract and shorten, is a unique property of muscle tissue. When a motor nerve innervates a muscle, that muscle contracts or shortens. If it is a skeletal muscle, the shortening moves the bones to which it is attached. The ability of muscles to shorten their length is essential to all movement. (See the next section for different types of contraction.)

- *Extensibility*—Extensibility is the ability of a muscle to stretch beyond its normal resting length. When a muscle stretches beyond its resting length, great flexibility and facilitation of movement are achieved. Extensibility is important for skeletal muscles, which often are stretched in warming up for more vigorous activity and prestretched before strength training routines.

- *Elasticity*—Elasticity is the ability of a muscle to rebound after being stretched. It is partly a function of the connective tissue within and surrounding muscle cells and groups of cells.

- *Tonicity*—Tonicity, or muscle tone or tonus, is a state of hardness or firmness of the main bulk of a muscle, known as the muscle belly. The greater the number of active muscle fibers and the less intramuscular fat, the firmer the muscle. *Muscle tone* is a more common term, and muscle tone is important aesthetically, as firm muscles are considered desirable. Muscle tone cannot be measured in a laboratory; instead, the perception of muscle tone is based on muscle hardness and a person's experience, knowledge, and judgment.

People often mistakenly believe that strength training to make muscles firmer and harder will result in fat loss. Working a muscle makes it firmer, harder, and stronger. It does not, however, reduce fat in the area around the muscle or turn fat into muscle. Aerobic/cardiovascular activity is more efficient in burning fat.

Different Types of Contraction

Contraction is a unique property of muscle cells (fibers), and several kinds of contraction can be identified. Anatomists traditionally refer to two types of contraction—isotonic and isometric.

■ *Isotonic contraction* occurs when a muscle changes in length upon contraction and movement takes place. An example of isotonic contraction is curling a 20-pound dumbbell. The elbow flexors are innervated and shorten, flexing the elbow. This action is called isotonic contraction of the elbow flexors. All movement, exercises, and activity involve the isotonic contraction of skeletal muscles.

■ *Isometric contraction* occurs when the muscle is innervated and contracts but does not change in length. Using the previous example of curling, suppose the dumbbell is too heavy for the person to curl. When the person tries to curl the dumbbell, all the available muscle fibers of the elbow flexor muscles are innervated and try to shorten, but they cannot create enough force to curl the weight. The muscle fibers are working maximally, but movement is prevented by the excessive weight. This is an isometric contraction of the elbow flexors.

Applied anatomists and kinesiologists interested in analyzing muscle movement found this traditional classification limiting. They developed a different classification of isotonic contractions to describe muscle action more definitively. They now referred to movement that shortens the muscle as a *concentric contraction*. In addition, research has shown that the tension within the muscle does not remain constant as the muscle shortens; the muscle tension changes throughout the range of motion. The term *eccentric contraction* is now used to describe a muscle that lengthens as it creates muscle tension. In our example of curls, 20 pounds were curled, resulting in elbow flexion (concentric contraction); now visualize slowly lowering the same dumbbell until the elbow is extended or straight. As gravity works to pull the dumbbell down, the antagonists (the triceps) do not need to contract to cause elbow extension—gravity will do it. To lower the dumbbell slowly (and resist gravity), however, the elbow flexors (the muscles that curled the dumbbell) must slowly relax, allowing the elbow to extend slowly. The elbow flexors that curled the elbow thus now also lengthen to allow the dumbbell to be lowered to its starting position in an eccentric contraction. Table 3.2 shows the classifications of contractions.

Table 3.2   Classification of Contractions

Anatomy	Type of contraction	Kinesiology
Isotonic	Muscle length shortens	Concentric
	Muscle length increases	Eccentric
Isometric	No change in muscle length	Static

Muscle Fiber

The muscle fiber (cell) is the basic structural and functional unit of the muscle. Muscles are made up of thousands of these fibers or strands, many of which run the length of the muscle. The muscle cell is a complicated organ that uses oxygen, metabolizes food, and produces waste; thus, the fiber contains many structures and substances. Nutrients, oxygen, carbon dioxide, and waste products pass through the muscle cell membrane.

The muscle fiber membrane is a very delicate structure. The strength of the muscle fiber comes from a sheath of connective tissue, which surrounds each fiber and runs along its length. This sheath of connective tissue is called *endomysium*. To make the total muscle even stronger, a group of muscle fibers (with their endomysium) are wrapped in another sheath of connective tissue, called *perimysium*, to form a bundle of muscle fibers. This bundle is called a primary bundle or a *fasciculus*. To increase the muscle strength, a group of these primary bundles is wrapped in still another perimysium, making a secondary bundle. Large muscles may have a third bundling, following the same principle. Finally, a sheath of connective tissue named *epimysium* covers the whole muscle. Thus, in addition to muscle fibers, a great deal of connective tissue exists within the muscle.

The microscopic anatomy of the individual muscle fiber lies within the muscle cell membrane (*sarcolemma*). Inside the membrane is the cytoplasm (*sarcoplasm*) in which all the intracellular structures and substances exist. One of the important structures in the muscle fiber is the myofibril. The myofibril is made up of structural protein (actin and myosin) that arranges itself in a structural pattern within the myofibril. This protein structure is called the *cytoskeleton*. The myofibril is a very small tubular structure that is divided into segments called *sarcomeres* by protein (actin) disks called *Z lines*. Z is the first letter of a German word for *between*, and one sarcomere is bordered by two Z lines. Z lines are living protein, and thin protein appendages (*actin* myofilaments) come out of each Z line and go into the sarcomere but do not meet. Thick protein myofilaments (*myosin*) lie between the actin filaments but do not fill the entire space between the Z lines. Actin and myosin lie parallel to each other, creating a pattern that allows different amounts of light to pass through. The differing amounts of light give the striated muscle its light and dark bands. Actin and myosin filaments are connected by small cross-bridges, and when certain chemical and mechanical changes occur, these filaments slide past each other, causing the two Z lines to move closer together. Although this process results in a very small shortening of the myofibril, when the shortening is multiplied by thousands of myofibrils and sarcomeres, the total muscle shortens (contracts).

Figure 3.19 shows a sequence of drawings, starting with a total muscle. First, a small section is enlarged, showing one muscle fiber. Next, one of the myofibrils within the muscle cell is enlarged, and the striations can be seen clearly. The myofibril pictured shows a sarcomere, shown with labeling of the various parts: Z lines, A band, I band, H zone. The tubelike myofibril is submicroscopically small. Inside the myofibril are the actin and myosin filaments (see the bottom of figure 3.19). When the muscle contracts, each sarcomere shortens as the two Z lines move together slightly due to the cross-bridges that attach the actin to the myosin filaments (the cross-bridges are not shown in figure 3.19). When the sarcomere shortens, the filaments slide over one another, causing the H zone either to disappear or to become very small; the same thing happens to the I band.

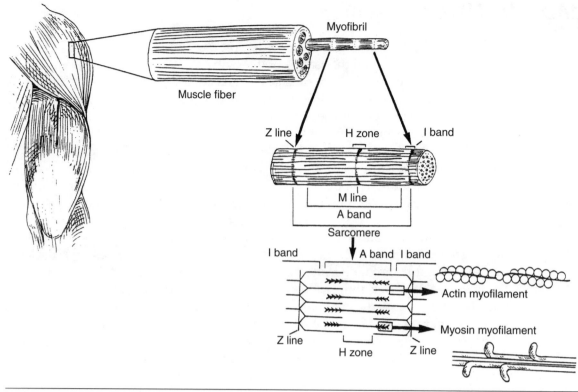

Figure 3.19 The muscle and its sections.

Muscle fibers come in several types, they work on an all-or-nothing principle, and they are innervated by motor units. These three important concepts are discussed in the following sections.

Muscle Fiber Types

All muscle cells are not the same. Because of their biochemical makeup, some are well suited for explosive, fast contraction and can do work without oxygen, although they fatigue quickly. These are the fast-twitch fibers, and they are recruited by the nervous system when sprinting, explosive activity is undertaken. When prolonged muscular activity is performed that requires the muscle fibers to work for a longer period of time without fatigue, a different type of muscle fiber is recruited, one that requires oxygen and resists fatigue. Such fibers are the slow-twitch fibers. All muscles contain both types of fibers, although some muscles have higher percentages of one kind of fiber over the other, making them more suitable for either endurance or sprinting activities.

Besides the basic two types of fast- and slow-twitch fibers, an intermediate type of fiber has also been identified. However, for our practical use it's enough to know the two types of muscle fibers, one used for prolonged work and the other for short, fast work. For a more complete understanding of muscle fiber typing, read some of the articles listed in the reading list on page 43.

All-or-None Principle

When a motor nerve innervates an individual muscle fiber, the fiber contracts (shortens); when the fiber contracts it does so either maximally or it does not contract at all. This theory of muscle contraction is called the "all-or-none" principle. Muscle fibers do not contract partially; however, a total muscle can partially contract. If one can maximally curl 100 pounds, then a 50-pound curl is half of the maximum contraction. This partial contraction is a result of a maximum contraction of only some muscle fibers, but the fibers in the total muscle that are contracted are maximally contracted.

To the biologist, the size or cross section area of a muscle is a reflection of the number of fibers and thus the total strength of the muscle. A muscle with twice the cross-sectional area of another muscle will be twice as strong as the other muscle. We do not have the use of all the muscle fibers that are available to us. When muscle fibers that we were born with have never been used, we can't use them until they are brought into play by continually stressing the muscle. So we can voluntarily recruit only a percentage of the fibers that are present. Rather than create more or new fibers, strength training brings into play fibers that are already there but have not been innervated because they have not been used. By consistently imposing an overload and stress or demand on the muscle, we can bring additional fibers into play, thus developing the strength of the total muscle.

Strength acquisition is training or bringing into play muscle fibers that are present but have not previously been able to be innervated voluntarily. *Maximal physiological strength* is achieved when all the available fibers can be contracted voluntarily.

In its most simple form, strength training is stressing the muscle to bring latent muscle fibers into play. By varying the kind of activity we engage in during strength training, we can present a stress or overload of the muscle that recruits both fast-twitch and slow-twitch muscle fibers.

Motor Units

A motor nerve innervates every muscle fiber, but a single nerve goes to many muscle fibers. The group of muscle fibers that is innervated by a single motor nerve is called a *motor unit*. When innervated, all muscle fibers in a unit contract maximally. The muscle fibers within a motor unit are all the same type of fiber— fast-twitch, slow-twitch, or intermediate.

Effects of Strength Training on Muscles

Strength training can make muscles grow in size, and pumping them up can make them look even larger. Working out generates lactic acid and may cause acute muscle soreness but not delayed-onset muscle soreness (DOMS). Contrary to myth, working out does not require exercisers to eat more protein.

Muscle Hypertrophy

Muscles can grow bigger (muscle hypertrophy), although within limits. Muscle hypertrophy results from the development of more blood capillaries within the muscle tissue, the enlargement of individual muscle fibers as a result of an increase in the amounts of chemicals and protein myofilaments within the cells, and the thickening of connective tissue around the muscle. Also, inactive fibers can become active and enlarge. The total result is muscle hypertrophy.

Although hypertrophy will occur as a response to strength training, a tall, thin individual will never develop the 22-in. biceps of a short, muscular person. We inherit our basic body type, or *somatotype*, and we cannot change it. Each of us falls into one of three basic body types:

- *Endomorphs*: Endomorphs have massive frames with large anterior and posterior diameters. This body type has a tendency to carry fat.
- *Mesomorphs*: Also called athletic types, mesomorphs have a triangular shape, with broad shoulders and narrow hips.
- *Ectomorphs*: Ectomorphs are tall and lean, with long bones.

Each body type can increase muscle and fat somewhat, but basically the body type stays the same.

Although muscles do become larger when trained, the before-and-after pictures in many muscle magazines are misleading. An underdeveloped mesomorph can make big changes when he or she trains because the body type permits it. A picture of Arnold Schwartzenegger at age 12 shows that he was a mesomorph before he dedicated himself to strength training.

Certainly we can add or take off fat, and with hard work we can increase muscle size. But our basic shape and contour is predetermined by heredity. The elite female bodybuilder is born with the body structure that will enable her, with hard training and discipline, to become a champion.

Muscle Pumping

Bodybuilders employ a technique of rapid and sustained muscle contractions known as the "pump up" to increase muscle size before posing. We all have experienced this each time we've had blood drawn from an arm. The laboratory technician tells you to make a fist strongly three or four times to make the veins in the forearm stand out. This is a mild form of pumping up. The conditioned skeletal muscle is very vascular (contains many blood vessels). By contracting the muscle and holding the contraction, we can pump blood into a muscle, causing it to enlarge. The increased blood flow within the muscle, however, does not go on indefinitely; the pumping has to be maintained continuously to keep the increase in size.

Lactic Acid

Lactic acid is a normal chemical byproduct of muscle metabolism. It accumulates in the muscles and blood when insufficient oxygen is available to break it down and remove it. If muscular contraction continues without oxygen, the lactate will build up until it prevents muscle fibers from contracting. As soon as exercise stops, the body hyperventilates, in part to provide oxygen to convert the accumulated lactic acid into water and carbon dioxide. The water and carbon dioxide are removed by the kidneys and lungs and expelled from the body. Excess lactic acid is usually totally removed 30 minutes after strenuous exercise. Contrary to popular belief, lactic acid does not remain in the muscles after exercise, and it does not cause delayed muscle soreness or muscle cramps.

Muscle Soreness

Virtually everyone who has exercised has suffered from muscle soreness. Several theories have been put forth about the reasons for muscle soreness, and only in the early 1990s has research shown the cause of this common complaint. First, two kinds of muscle soreness exist: acute muscle soreness and delayed onset muscle soreness (DOMS). Acute muscle soreness occurs when a muscle is used repeatedly and soreness develops in that muscle. After the exercise stops, the soreness goes away quickly. If the muscle soreness starts 24 to 48 hours after exercise, however, it is considered to be DOMS. Earlier in this chapter we discussed the protein makeup of the muscle cell (myofibril, actin, and myosin protein filaments). These structures are termed the *cytoskeleton* of the muscle fiber. Priscilla Clarkson from the University of Massachusetts has shown that in DOMS this cytoskeleton is disrupted, causing swelling and the accumulation of white blood cells to sensitize the sensory nerve receptors in the muscle fibers, resulting in pain. This type of soreness typically follows severe eccentric contraction of the muscle.

Muscle Protein

The muscle contains a number of structural proteins, and the contractile elements of the muscle are made of proteins (actin and myosin filaments). We cannot obtain these proteins from foods. Strength training enthusiasts often believe that supplementary protein is necessary for muscle hypertrophy, muscle strength, and muscle training, and some muscle magazines have capitalized on this false belief.

Adequate protein intake is essential to all humans. Proteins are broken down into 23 amino acids required by the body, which often are referred to as the building blocks of protein. An amino acid pool exists from which structured protein is formed. Even if we eat no protein at all, however, the liver can make 15 of the amino acids (proteins) that we need. The liver cannot manufacture eight of these amino acids without protein, so these must come from the diet. The amino acids that must come from the diet are known as the *essential amino acids,* and they are readily available in meat (and poultry and fish), eggs, and dairy products (milk, butter, cheese, ice cream).

The terms *complete* and *incomplete protein* are based on the essential amino acids. A complete protein contains all eight essential amino acids; an incomplete protein does not. Most vegetable protein is incomplete, so vegetable protein must be eaten in combinations (e.g., legumes and seeds) that ensure that all eight amino acids are ingested during a day. If all eight amino acids are not eaten within the day, the formation of structural protein is compromised.

An adult needs approximately .75 grams of protein per kilogram of body weight. For example, a 170-pound man (77 kilograms) needs 58 grams of protein a day, which is easily obtainable in the average well-planned diet. Little evidence exists that an athlete needs more protein than do individuals who don't exercise. In addition, excess protein must be specially treated in the body and excreted by the kidneys. Excess protein can be damaging to the kidneys if an individual does not consume sufficient amounts of water.

Reading List

Heyward, Vivian H. 1998. *Advanced fitness assessment and exercise prescription.* Champaign, IL: Human Kinetics.

McArdle, William D., Frank I. Katch, and Victor L. Katch. 1991. *Exercise physiology. Energy, nutrition, and human performance*. Philadelphia: Lea & Febiger.

Nieman, David C. 1995. *Fitness and sports medicine. A health-related approach*. Palo Alto, CA: Bull.

Plowman, Sharon A., and Denise L. Smith. 1997. *Exercise physiology for health, fitness, and performance*. Boston, MA: Allyn & Bacon.

Powers, Scott K. and Edward T. Howley. 1997. *Exercise physiology. Theory and application to fitness and performance*. Chicago, IL: Brown and Benchmark.

Answers to Muscle Action Quiz (Page 34)

1. Head or neck flexors
2. Head or neck extensors, resulting in hyperextension of neck
3. Arm or shoulder flexors
4. Arm or shoulder extensors
5. Arm or shoulder adductors
6. Shoulder (arm) flexors and elbow flexors
7. Elbow extensors (arm in flexed position)
8. Knee flexors
9. Knee extensors
10. Hip (leg) flexors and knee flexors
11. Hip or leg extensors, resulting in hyperextension of hip
12. Hip or leg adductors
13. Hip or leg abductors

Selected Muscle Groups

Wrist Flexion

Flexor carpi radialis
Flexor carpi ulnaris
Flexor digitorum longus
Flexor digitorum profundus
Flexor digitorum sublimus
Flexor pollicis longus
Palmaris longus

Wrist Extension

Extensor carpi radialis brevis
Extensor carpi radialis longus
Extensor carpi ulnaris
Extensor digitorum communis

Elbow Flexion

Biceps brachii
Brachialis
Brachioradialis
Flexor digitorum sublimus
Pronator teres
Supinator

Elbow Extension

Anconeus
Extensor digitorum communis
Triceps

Radial-Ulna Pronation
Pronator teres
Pronator quadratus

Radial-Ulna Supination
Biceps brachii
Brachioradialis
Supinator

Shoulder Flexion
Anterior deltoid
Biceps brachii
Coracobrachialis
Pectoralis major

Shoulder Extension
Latissimus dorsi
Posterior deltoid
Teres major
Teres minor
Triceps

Shoulder Abduction
Infraspinatus (upper fibers)
Middle deltoid
Supraspinatus

Shoulder Adduction
Coracobrachialis
Infraspinatus
Latissimus dorsi
Pectoralis major
Teres major
Teres minor
Triceps

Shoulder Inward Rotation
Anterior deltoid
Latissimus dorsi
Pectoralis major
Subscapularis
Teres major

Shoulder Outward Rotation
Infraspinatus
Posterior deltoid
Teres minor

Neck Flexion
Sternocleidomastoid

Neck Extension
Splenius capitus
Trapezius

Neck Rotation
Sternocleidomastoid
Splenius capitus

Spine Flexion
External abdominal oblique
Internal abdominal oblique
Rectus abdominis

Spine Extension
Erector spinae (sacrospinalis)
Quadratus lumborum
Splenius capitus

Neck Lateral Flexion
Sternocleidomastoid
Splenius capitus

Spine Lateral Flexion
Iliocostalis lumborum
Quadratus lumborum

Hip Flexion

Adductor brevis
Adductor longus
Adductor magnus
Gluteus medius (anterior fibers)
Gluteus minimus (anterior fibers)
Gracilis
Iliacus
Pectineus
Psoas
Rectus femorus
Sartorius
Tensor fascia latae

Hip Extension

Adductor magnus (lower fibers)
Biceps femoris
Gluteus maximus
Gluteus medius (posterior fibers)
Gluteus minimus (posterior fibers)
Semimembranosis
Semitendinosis

Hip Abduction

Gluteus minimus
Gluteus medius
Gluteus maximus (superior fibers)
Sartorius
Tensor fascia latae

Hip Adduction

Adductor brevis
Adductor longus
Adductor magnus (lower fibers)
Biceps femoris
Gluteus maximus (deep fibers)
Gracilis
Pectineus
Psoas
Semimembranosis
Semitendinosis
Iliacus

Inward Rotation of the Hip

Adductor magnus (lower fibers)
Gluteus minimus (anterior fibers)
Gluteus medius (anterior fibers)
Semimembranosis
Semitendinosis
Tensor fascia latae

Outward Rotation of the Hip

Adductor brevis
Adductor longus
Adductor magnus (upper fibers)
Biceps femoris
Gluteus medius (posterior fibers)
Gluteus minimus (posterior fibers)
Iliacus
Pectineus
Psoas
Sartorius

Knee Flexion

Biceps femoris
Gastrocnemius
Gracilis
Sartorius
Semimembranosis
Semitendinosis

Knee Extension

Rectus femoris
Vastus intermedius
Vastus lateralis
Vastus medialis

Plantar Flexion

Flexor digitorum longus
Flexor hallicus longus
Gastrocnemius
Peroneus brevis
Peroneus longus
Plantaris
Soleus
Tibialis posterior

Dorsal Flexion

Extensor digitorum longus
Extensor hallicus longus
Peroneus tertius
Tibialis anterior

Inversion

Flexor hallicus longus
Tibialis anterior
Tibialis posterior

Eversion

Peroneus brevis
Peroneus longus
Peroneus tertius

Chapter 4

The Cardiorespiratory System

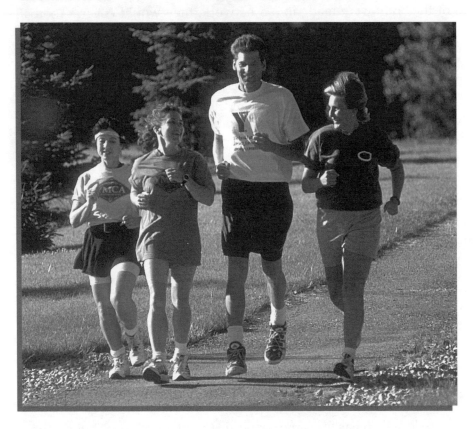

The cardiorespiratory system consists of the heart, lungs, and circulation. *Cardiovascular* refers to the heart and circulation; however, because oxygen comes from the air surrounding us, the respiratory system is also intimately involved with the circulatory system, which transports the oxygen to the tissues of the body.

Cardiovascular System

Blood vessels carrying blood away from the heart are called *arteries*, and smaller arteries are called *arterioles*. Blood vessels carrying blood toward the heart are called *veins*, and smaller veins are called *venules*. These vessels are muscular-walled conduits that transport the blood rapidly to the various parts of the body. The blood moves so quickly through these relatively large conduits that a considerable volume of blood is not even in contact with the walls of the arteries and veins.

Blood is the transportation system of the body—anything that is going somewhere in the body is transported there by the blood. Once the blood arrives at its destination, however, the arteriole wall is too thick to pass through the body tissue. Passing substances from the blood to the tissue is the job of the *capillaries,* which lie between the arterioles and the venules. The capillaries are the real working part of the circulatory system where the exchange between substances in the blood and the tissue takes place. Several factors facilitate their task:

- The number of capillaries is very great. Many junior high school health education textbooks try to impress their readers by showing that if all the capillaries of the body were made into a network, they would cover a football field.

- The capillaries have extremely small diameters so that virtually everything in the blood moving through them is in contact with the capillary walls. The small diameter facilitates an exchange between the tissue and the blood.

- The walls of the capillaries are microscopically thin, allowing substances that are being carried by the blood to pass through the capillary walls to the surrounding tissue and substances in the surrounding tissue to enter the capillaries.

- Blood moves very slowly through the capillaries, allowing time for the exchange between the substances in the blood and the surrounding cells to take place.

The heart is the pump that keeps blood moving through the cardiovascular system. We take a look at how it works, define some related terms, and discuss heart sounds. Then we turn to a discussion of blood pressure, how it's measured, and how it relates to exercise. Next, we talk about heart rate—how to count heart rate, what steady-state and maximum heart rate are, and how heart rate relates to work done during exercise. Last, we examine the components of blood and blood's capacity to carry oxygen to muscles when needed during exercise.

Heart Muscle

The heart muscle, which has the same properties as all muscles, is about the size of a large fist. It is located in the center of the chest just behind the sternum, and it is tilted slightly to the left so that the apex of the heart is to the left of the lower sternum. The heart is a hollow muscle with the myocardium (the belly of the muscle) surrounding the hollow interior. The inside of the heart is divided by walls into four chambers, two above and two below (see figure 4.1). The two upper chambers, the left and right atrium, receive the blood and pump it to the two lower chambers, the right and left ventricle, which then eject the blood out of the heart. A wall in anatomy is called a *septum,* so that the wall that separates the left and right atria is called the *interatrial septum.* The wall between the ventricles is called the *interventricular septum.* The wall between the atria and the ventricles is called the *atrioventricular septum.*

This terminology allows one to identify parts of the heart. The atrial myocardium, for example, is the heart muscle surrounding the atria, the ventricular myocardium is the muscle that surrounds the ventricles, and the right ventricular myocardium is the muscle surrounding the right ventricle. An electrocardio-

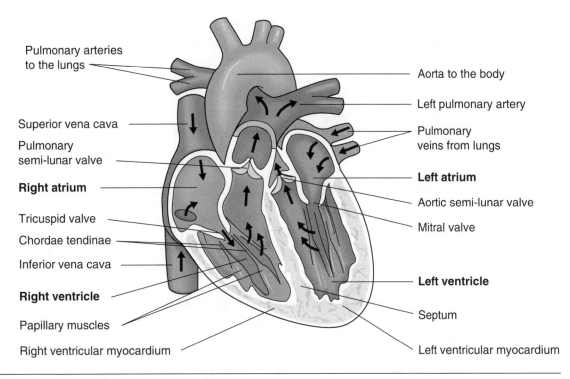

Figure 4.1 The heart.

gram condition exists called LVH or left ventricular hypertrophy. Familiarity with the terminology allows you to understand this condition quickly: it is hypertrophy (muscle enlargement) of the heart muscle surrounding the left ventricle.

The heart is a reciprocating pump. It fills and ejects, and blood pressure and one-way valves control the direction of the blood. Figure 4.1 shows schematically the circulation of the blood through the heart. All of the blood from the lower extremities and the lower trunk returns to the heart through larger and larger venules and veins until it finally arrives at the heart in a large vein called the inferior vena cava. This vein delivers the blood into the upper right hand chamber, the right atrium. Likewise all of the blood from the upper extremities, the head, and upper trunk also returns to the heart through larger and larger venules and veins, finally becoming the superior vena cava, which also delivers the blood into the upper right-hand chamber.

When the heart beats (contracts), first the upper chambers contract and then the lower chambers contract. Then the upper chambers relax and finally the lower chambers relax. This cycle is one heartbeat. It is easier to discuss the heart as two separate pumps (which it is), the right side of the heart and the left side of the heart. When the upper chambers contract, the blood is pushed from the upper chambers to the lower chambers. On the right side there are two possible places for the blood to go:

- The blood could go back from whence it came, but this is prevented by venous blood pressure forcing blood into the heart and also by the one-way valves in veins that prevent the blood from changing direction.
- The blood can pass through a large valve (the tricuspid valve) that leads to the lower right chamber, the right ventricle.

Similarly, looking at the left-hand side of the heart, blood that has left the lungs and entered the upper-left chamber through the pulmonary veins is pushed out of the chamber by the contraction. As on the right side, the blood has the same two choices; and, like the right-hand side, it passes through a large valve (the mitral or bicuspid valve) to the lower-left chamber, the left ventricle. When the lower chambers contract, they do so forcefully, ejecting the blood out of the ventricles. Because the tricuspid and mitral valves are one-way flutter valves, they prevent the blood from going back to the upper chambers. The blood within the ventricles is forcefully ejected through valves into large blood vessels leaving the heart. On the right side the blood passes through the pulmonary semilunar valve into the pulmonary artery and sends the blood to the lungs. On the left-hand side the blood passes through the aortic semilunar valve into the aorta and sends the blood to all parts of the body.

The heart is really two pumps that are joined together. No connection exists between the right and left side of the heart except through the lungs.

All of the blood leaves the right ventricle, moves through the pulmonary arteries to the lungs, and returns to the left side of the heart through the pulmonary veins. This circuit is known as *pulmonary circulation.* In a similar fashion, all of the blood leaves the left ventricle and goes through the aorta to all parts of the body (running through all systems, such as the respiratory system, the muscular system, and the nervous system). It then returns to the heart through the superior and inferior vena cavas. Because the blood is going to all the body systems in this part of the circuit it is called *systemic circulation* (see figure 4.2).

Neither pulmonary circulation nor systemic circulation supplies the myocardium (the heart muscle) with blood, so the heart has its own circulation. Starting with two large coronary arteries arising from the aorta as it leaves the heart, the blood is delivered to the myocardium through coronary arteries, capillaries, and veins. This system is called *coronary circulation,* and it is most important because it includes the arteries that are involved in coronary heart disease (see figure 4.3).

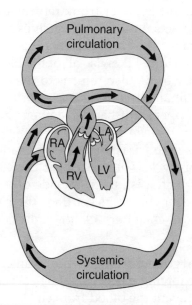

Figure 4.2 Pulmonary and systemic circulation.

The Cardiorespiratory System ■ 53

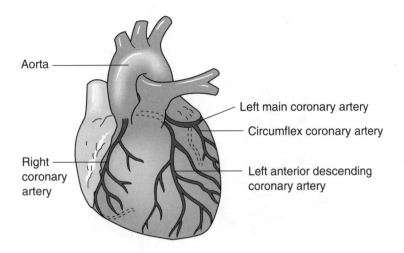

Figure 4.3 Coronary circulation.

Here are definitions for some terms used in discussing the heart. Some of these terms are illustrated in figure 4.4.

- *Ischemia.* Ischemia means lack of blood flow. It can occur in any part of the body. If the lack of blood flow is to the myocardium, this is known as *myocardial ischemia.*

- *Angina pectoris.* Angina pectoris is chest pains resulting from myocardial ischemia. Angina is a symptom of coronary insufficiency. The heart at rest is very efficient, so even some narrowing of the coronary artery often causes no discomfort or symptoms. When exercise, however, causes the heart to beat faster because more blood (and oxygen) is needed to do the added work, any narrowing causes myocardial ischemia and pain. This pain is very symptomatic and is felt under the sternum, down the left arm, and often up to the jaw on the left-hand side. A typical anginal attack involves these symptoms, warning the individual of pending disaster.

- *Thrombosis.* Thrombosis is a blood clot in a blood vessel. A blood clot in the coronary artery is a *coronary thrombosis.*

- *Infarction.* Infarction is the death of cells, which are usually replaced with scar tissue. *Myocardial infarction* is the death of heart muscle cells due to a lack of oxygen. The extent to which the left ventricle is affected determines whether the myocardial infarction is fatal or nonfatal. Myocardial infarction (MI) is written on more death certificates in the United States than any other cause of death. The American Heart Association indicates that millions of nonfatal heart attacks occur each year without the individual knowing. These "silent heart attacks" are often dismissed as indigestion and will only show up on an electrocardiogram (EKG) at a later date.

- *Pulmonary.* Pulmonary refers to the lungs. The pulmonary arteries and veins, respectively, take blood to and from the lungs. A pulmonary function laboratory in a hospital tests lung function.

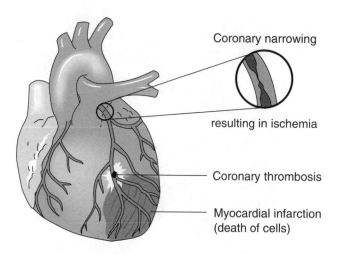

Figure 4.4 Ischemia, thrombosis, and infarction.

The familiar "lub-dub" sound heard through the stethoscope is the sound of the closing of the tricuspid and mitral valves and the blood as it passes through the semilunar valves of the heart (see figure 4.5). The physician can diagnose valve and blood flow problems in the heart by listening to a patient's heart sounds. The stethoscope is used by fitness directors to count heart rate during exercise, but for the physician it is a diagnostic instrument. The two sounds ("lub" and "dub") that are heard at rest become one sound when the heart rate approaches 100 beats per minute (beats/min).

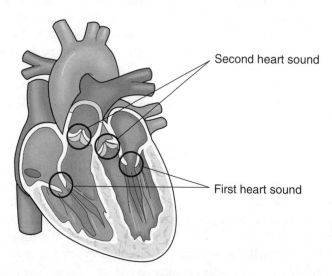

Figure 4.5 Heart sounds.

Blood Pressure

Any time fluid flows through a pipe or tube, it exerts pressure on the walls of the pipe. The faster it is pumped through the pipe, the greater the pressure it exerts on the pipe walls. Similarly, blood passing through the arteries and veins exerts a pressure on the walls of these vessels; this is called *blood pressure*. As one exercises and the heart beats faster (pumping more blood through the arteries and veins), blood pressure increases. The elevated blood pressure is a natural result of exercising. Blood pressure must increase; the harder you work, the higher the blood pressure. Figure 4.6 shows that with increasing amounts of work, the systolic blood pressure (SBP) rises and the diastolic blood pressure (DBP) stays the same or may rise a little and then level off. The difference between SBP and DBP is called pulse pressure, which must get larger when work is increased.

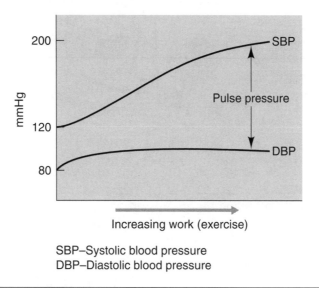

Figure 4.6 Exercise and blood pressure.

Blood pressure is a very common measurement for fitness directors and exercise physiologists to take. It is one of the few medical tests that those in the medical community do not mind nonmedical persons performing. It is simple to take accurately, and, because the medical profession would like people to know their blood pressure levels, it encourages nonphysicians to monitor blood pressure. High blood pressure, also called hypertension, is often referred to as "the silent killer" because it has few symptoms; in fact, individuals who have high blood pressure often are not aware of the problem.

Figure 4.7 illustrates taking blood pressure with a mercury sphygmomanometer. Although this is a simple technique, it bears explaining. The subject sits upright in a straight-backed chair with both feet flat on the floor. His or her arm rests on a table or platform so that the elbow is flexed at about 100°. The blood pressure cuff is a nylon sleeve wrapped around a rubber bladder, much like a small bicycle inner tube. The person taking the measurement wraps the cuff and the bladder snugly around the subject's upper left arm, leaving about an inch between the bottom of the cuff and the inside surface of the elbow (antecubital space). The cuff should be at heart level. Like a bicycle inner tube, the cuff can be inflated using a small pump in the form of a rubber ball. As the cuff inflates, it gets tighter around the arm, creating a tourniquet around the upper arm and stopping the blood flow in the brachial artery.

After a few pumps, a tire pressure gauge tells you the pressure in a bicycle inner tube in pounds per square inch (psi). Likewise, the mercury column of the sphygmomanometer is the gauge that reflects the pressure in the cuff, which is measured in millimeters of mercury (mmHg). Usually the cuff is inflated to a

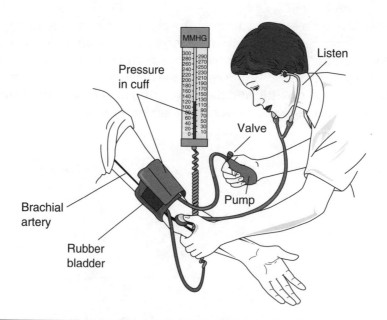

Figure 4.7 Indirect method of taking blood pressure.

pressure of 200 mmHg, which will stop the blood flow in the brachial artery in most people (except those with high blood pressure). The person taking the blood pressure then places the stethoscope in the antecubital space and opens the escape valve (the little chrome knob next to the rubber ball) to slowly release the air in the cuff. While the air is slowly being released, the mercury in the column slowly decreases in height, reflecting the decreasing pressure in the cuff. The mercury drops slowly but steadily at about 2 mmHg per second, which means the mercury will be dropping for about 75 seconds (approximately a 150-mmHg drop from 200 mmHg to about 50 mmHg). The person taking the blood pressure listens with the stethoscope. At some point as the pressure decreases, the blood dammed up in the brachial artery behind the tourniquet has enough pressure to pass under the cuff and start flowing to the lower arm. When this occurs, the stethoscope will pick up the sound of the blood escaping under the cuff. It will sound just like the heartbeat. The moment the sound is detected, without stopping the release of the pressure in the cuff, the person taking the blood pressure takes a reading of the height of the mercury. He or she continues to slowly release the pressure in the cuff and to monitor the sound until it disappears. The moment the sound disappears, the person takes another reading of the height of the mercury. The subject's blood pressure has now been taken, and it is reported as the height of the mercury column when the sound was first heard and the height of the mercury column when the sound disappeared. The moment the sound disappears, the rest of the pressure can be released from the cuff. If the first or second sound is missed, the person taking the blood pressure should not immediately pump the cuff up again; instead, he or she should release the pressure completely and repeat the measurement after a short rest.

The method of taking blood pressure just described is called the indirect method of taking blood pressure. It is indirect because it did not directly measure the pressure of the blood but instead the pressure of the cuff. From that information we extrapolated that the cuff pressure was also the pressure in the artery. A textbook normal blood pressure reading for an adult is 120/80, which is 120 mmHg/

80 mmHg. Using this example of 120/80, when the cuff pressure was 120 mmHg and the blood pushing under the cuff to the lower arm was heard, the force (pressure) of the blood must also have been 120 mmHg to get through the cuff's restriction. Likewise, when the cuff no longer restricted blood flow and the blood flowed freely under the cuff, the sound of the pumping disappeared.

The stage of the heartbeat cycle in which the heart contracts and ejects blood is called the heart's *systole*, so the pressure resulting from the ejected blood is called *systolic blood pressure* (SBP). The stage of the heartbeat cycle in which the heart is relaxed and is filling with blood is called the *diastole*, so the pressure resulting from the heart filling with blood is called *diastolic blood pressure* (DBP).

As the heart beats faster during exercise, systolic blood pressure rises steadily with increased work. Diastolic blood pressure may rise a little and then plateau. The difference between systolic and diastolic blood pressure is called *pulse pressure*. Pulse pressure must increase during progressive exercise (see figure 4.6 on page 55).

Normal adult resting systolic blood pressure is usually between 110 and 125 mmHg, and diastolic blood pressure is 80 mmHg or less. When someone's systolic pressure is between 125 and about 140 mmHg and/or the diastolic pressure is 80 to 90 mmHg, the person is said to have *borderline hypertension*. When a person's systolic pressure is above 140 mmHg and the diastolic pressure is over 90 mmHg, he or she is said to have *hypertension*.

Figure 4.8 shows the brachial pulse wave, which is a tracing that comes from the blood as it passes under the blood pressure cuff. Each time the heart beats the brachial wave rises, then drops between beats in the pattern shown. Some exercise testing machines track these waves to count heart rate.

As blood pressure normally increases with exercise, individuals with uncontrolled high blood pressure should not exercise vigorously because their blood pressure will rise above safe limits. In hypertensive exercisers, blood pressure should be controlled or the exercise intensity should be kept low.

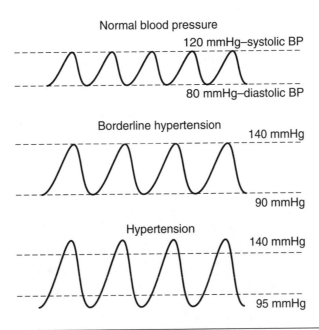

Figure 4.8 Blood pressure shown by the brachial pulse wave.

Two types of sphygmomanometers exist: the mercury sphygmomanometer just described and an aneroid sphygmomanometer, which contains no mercury. Because mercury is classified as a hazardous substance (mercury vapor is poisonous, and mercury itself is very difficult to clean up), mercury sphygmomanometers are usually used only in laboratories, hospitals, or doctor's offices and are typically attached to a wall. Portable blood pressure devices are aneroid sphygmomanometers. They are very accurate and are calibrated against mercury sphygmomanometers (see figure 4.9).

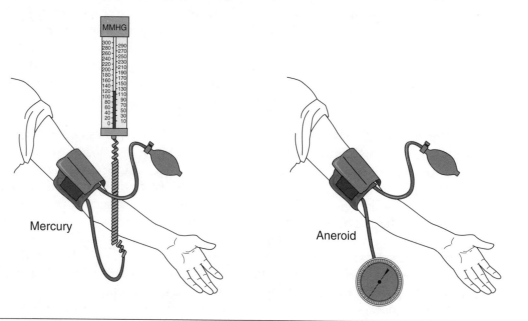

Figure 4.9 Types of sphygmomanometers.

Heart Rate

Fitness testers have been measuring heart rate (or pulse rate) to assess cardiorespiratory fitness from the time fitness testing first began. Heart rate is usually reported as beats per minute (beats/min). Here are three principles relating to heart rate that have been used for cardiorespiratory testing:

■ *Principle 1. The lower the resting heart rate, the fitter the person.* This concept is only a principle, not an absolute. An individual may have a low or high resting heart rate for many other reasons besides fitness. We know that cardiovascular athletes have low resting heart rates, assuming that the athlete is normal and has no pathology. It has been shown hundreds of times that as an individual improves her or his cardiorespiratory fitness, her or his resting heart rate goes down. The following are general heart rate ranges:

    a. Normal resting heart rate   50–100 beats/min

    b. Average resting heart rate   72 beats/min

    c. An aerobically fit person   50–65 beats/min*

    d. An aerobically fit athlete   40–50 beats/min*

* Ranges *c* and *d* are approximations, as there is a wide range of aerobically fit individuals as well as a wide range of cardiovascular elite athletes.

■ *Principle 2. The lower an individual's exercise heart rate, the more aerobically fit she or he is.* Assuming a group of individuals is doing the same amount of work, the lower the exercise heart rate, the fitter the person. If 20 people were riding a cycle ergometer 600 kg per minute, then the individual whose heart rate increased the least would be considered the fittest. Obviously there are exceptions, but as a general principle this rule is true.

■ *Principle 3. After exercise, the quicker the heart rate returns to its pre-exercise rate, the fitter the person.* All the early step tests were based on this principle, as all of them used the recovery heart rate to determine an individual's fitness level.

Counting the Heart Rate

Several methods can be used to determine one's heart rate:

- Count the number of heartbeats for 60 seconds.
- Count the number of heartbeats for 15 seconds and multiply by 4.
- Count the number of heartbeats for 10 seconds and multiply by 6.
- Count the number of heartbeats for 6 seconds and multiply by 10.

All these methods will result in the number of heartbeats per minute. Any time a count is multiplied, however, any error in counting (even by as much as a half beat) is also multiplied. For example, if you count the heart rate for 6 seconds, get 7, and multiply it by 10, then the heart rate is 70 beats/min. But as we only count in whole numbers, what if the count were actually 7.7? Then the heart rate would really be 77 beats/min.

To get an accurate resting heart rate, the best method is to count for a full 60 seconds to avoid multiplication errors. Methods that count for less than a minute are usually used to determine the exercise heart rate by counting the heart rate after stopping exercise. When you stop exercising, your heart rate recovers very quickly, so if you're trying to estimate your exercise heart rate, the quicker you can take the heart rate and the shorter the time period between stopping exercise and taking the measurement, the better the estimate.

In the YMCA cycle ergometer test, the exercise heart rate is measured while the person is exercising. To get the most accurate reading the heart rate is monitored using a stethoscope. Locate the place on the chest where the heartbeat is loudest and then, when the person monitoring is ready to count, he or she times 30 beats with a stopwatch. The slower the heart rate, the longer it takes the person's heart to beat 30 times; the faster the heart rate, the shorter the 30 beats take.

Counting should start on zero, as a cycle is being measured. The first beat is the start of the cycle; one beat later is one heartbeat. Counting heartbeats from zero is analogous to when an infant is born. At birth the infant is not one year old; only a year later is that infant one year old.

The method of timing 30 beats is used in the YMCA test, so it is important for you to understand the basis of its use. Although a conversion table is included in this book (table 6.12, page 148), as a physical fitness tester you should know the formula on which the table is based (see figure 4.10).

Example (a) in figure 4.10 shows that the 30 beats took 10 seconds. If 30 beats took 10 seconds, the heart rate is 3 beats per second (30/10 = 3). Multiplying the beats per second by 60 will give beats per minute.

COUNTING H.R. - PWC max.

Time 30 beats >>> from table 6.12 >> get HR

Formula = $\dfrac{30}{\text{Time (sec)}}$ × 60 = bpm

OR

$\dfrac{30 \text{ seconds}}{\text{Time for the 30 beats}}$ = beats/sec × 60 = bpm

Examples:

a. 10sec. Calc.: $\dfrac{30}{10\text{sec}}$ = 3 beats/sec × 60 = 180 bpm

b. 14sec. Calc.: $\dfrac{30}{14\text{sec}}$ = 2.143 bps × 60 = 128 bpm

c. 20sec. Calc.: $\dfrac{30}{20\text{sec}}$ = 1.5 bps × 60 = 90 bpm

Not in the table

d. 30sec. Calc.: $\dfrac{30}{30\text{sec}}$ = 1 bps × 60 = 60 bpm

Figure 4.10 Timing 30 beats to get heart rate.

Steady-State Heart Rate

The moment an individual starts to work, her or his heart rate increases immediately. If the heart rate were taken at the end of the first minute it would be meaningless, as the heart rate would still be increasing. It takes *about* three minutes of exercise before the heart rate stabilizes. Once the heart rate plateaus it has reached what is called the *steady-state heart rate* (SSHR). SSHR represents the heart rate for a particular workload (see figure 4.11). Although SSHR usually occurs in about three minutes, it may take four or five minutes. Many European researchers wait six minutes to ensure SSHR.

If the difference between the second-minute heart rate and the third-minute heart rate is more than five beats/min, the heart rate is still increasing significantly, and a fourth or even a fifth minute should be added. When the difference in heart rate between the second and third minute (or between the third and fourth or fourth and fifth minutes) is five beats/min or less, it can be assumed that the heart rate has stabilized and SSHR has been attained. When the workload is increased, the same sequence of events occurs to establish an SSHR at the new, increased workload (see fig. 4.11).

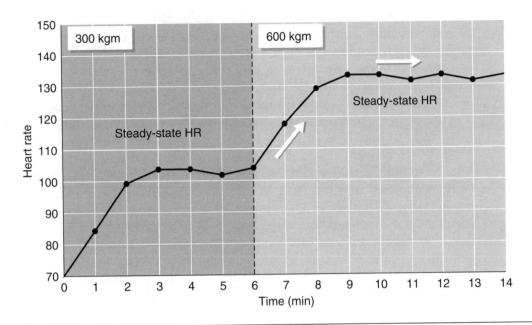

Figure 4.11 Steady-state heart rate.

Maximum Heart Rate

As an individual works harder, her or his heart rate increases linearly. The higher the workload, the higher the heart rate. At some point, however, even though the amount of work increases, the heart rate will not increase. This state of plateau is not considered to be an SSHR; at this point the heart has reached its fastest rate or *maximum heart rate* (see figure 4.12).

Note that each heart-rate plot point in figure 4.12 is an SSHR. To obtain that plot point (e.g., 300 kgm = 110 beats/min) the subject had to have worked for at least three minutes. Everyone has a workload at which the heart rate will go no

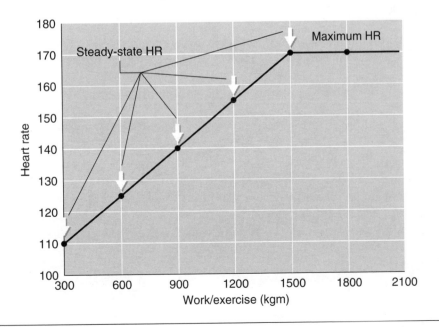

Figure 4.12 Maximum heart rate.

higher, and they have thus reached their maximum heart rate; this point, however, differs among individuals due to various reasons. The main reasons for the limitation of maximum heart rate are age and sedentary living (which usually accompanies aging). As one ages, the ability to drive the heart to high rates decreases. This decrease in maximum heart rate is generally accepted as a function of age, but it is also due to a decrease in physical fitness. In the general population this decrease in maximum heart rate is very evident. In individuals who are aerobically fit and who continue to exercise into later life the decrease is less dramatic, and the maximum heart rate decreases at a much slower rate.

In the general unfit population, maximum heart rate decreases with age linearly as depicted in figure 4.13. The formula of 220 minus an individual's age predicts that individual's maximum heart rate. For example, a 40-year-old male would have a predicted maximum heart rate of 180 (220 – 40 = 180). This prediction is only representative of the average 40-year-old male and does not take into account individual variations. Some 40-year-olds will have maximum heart rates higher or lower than 180 beats/min, but 180 beats/min is a good estimate.

In several studies a large number of subjects worked on a treadmill or cycle ergometer until maximum heart rate was obtained. Then an average maximum heart rate was calculated for each age group, based on the average of a distribution of scores for that age group. Figure 4.13 shows the results of one study that determined the average maximum heart rate of individuals between the ages of 20 and 70.

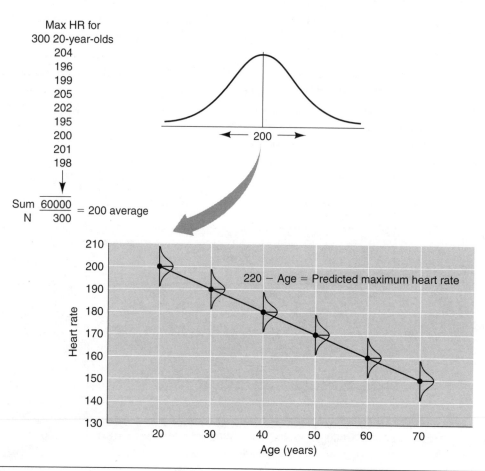

Figure 4.13 Maximum heart rate and age.

The upper left column of figure 4.13 shows the actual maximum heart rates for some of the 300 20-year-old subjects. Their maximum heart rates were added to get 60,000 and then were divided by 300 to arrive at the average maximum heart rate for 20-year-olds of 200 beats/min. These 300 scores were plotted to form a normal distribution of the scores with a mean of 200. See the normal distribution curve at the top of figure 4.13.

In the bottom graph of figure 4.13, maximum heart rate is plotted against age. The maximum heart rate for 20-year-olds of 200 is really the distribution curve lying on its side because some 20-year-olds were above or below the mean. The normal distribution curve for maximum heart rate was then plotted for each age group studied. Then the means of each distribution were joined to form the line showing the decrease in maximum heart rate with age.

Heart Rate and Work

As we saw earlier (figure 4.12), a linear relationship exists between work and heart rate. That linearity ends, however, when maximum heart rate is reached, and the maximum heart rate reached is based on age. Therefore the relationship between heart rate and work is only linear up to the point of maximum heart rate.

In like manner, at very low heart rates linearity may not exist because the heart rate can be affected by external stimuli. Say a man has a resting heart rate of 70 beats/min and rides the cycle ergometer at a low workload of 150 kgm. His heart rate increases to only 90 beats/min. This individual is not working very hard and therefore his heart is not working hard. If someone now tells a joke and the man begins to laugh, the laughter may increase his heart rate. Similar effects on heart rate can result from apprehension, nervousness, or any other external stimuli. By the time the heart rate gets to *about* 110 beats/min, however, it appears that external stimuli have a minimal effect on heart rate because now the heart is beating under the stress of exercise.

Two limitations exist therefore in the linear relationship between heart rate and work: maximum heart rate and heart rates below 110 beats/min. Figure 4.14 illustrates the linearity between heart rate and work and the exceptions.

Figure 4.15 shows the linearity between heart rate and work without the exceptions just mentioned. Although a linear relationship between heart rate and work can be observed, it does not follow necessarily that everyone has the same line. Figure 4.16 shows five individuals, all with a linear relationship between heart rate and work but all with different lines. The purpose of the cycle ergometer test is to determine this line for the person being tested.

The linear relationship allows one to predict a heart rate for any workload, or, conversely, one can predict the corresponding workload for any exercise heart rate. Sjostrand performed one of the early tests that used the linear relationship to predict maximum workload. Sjostrand worked with male iron ore factory workers in Central Europe and wanted to determine their working capacity. Sjostrand conducted this study in the days prior to the 220 − age formula for predicting maximum heart rate. He chose a heart rate of 170 beats/min as the assumed maximum heart rate for the individuals participating in his study. Assuming 170 beats/min as the maximum heart rate for his subjects, he wanted to determine how much work they could do if they worked maximally (which was 170 beats/min). Each subject was tested on a cycle ergometer. A low workload was imposed, and after six minutes an SSHR was counted. A second workload

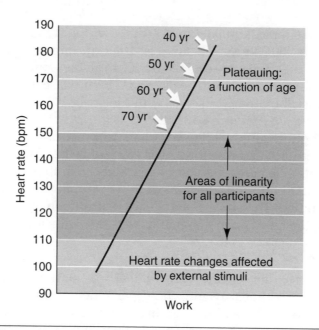

Figure 4.14 Linear relationship between heart rate and work, with exceptions.

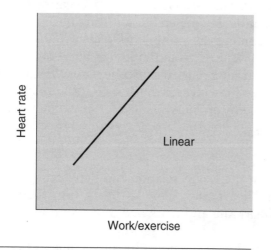

Figure 4.15 Linearity between work and heart rate, without exceptions.

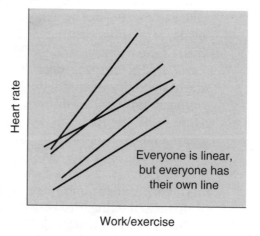

Figure 4.16 Five individuals all with linear relationship between heart rate and work.

was imposed that was slightly higher, and after another six minutes the second SSHR was counted (see figure 4.17). Because it was accepted in the scientific literature that a linear relationship existed between heart rate and work, all Sjostrand needed to establish that line was two SSHRs. These two plot points were then joined and extrapolated to the assumed maximum heart rate of 170 beats/min. As Sjostrand had established for that subject the line between heart rate and workload, he could then predict that if the subject had actually cycled to a heart rate of 170, he would have been doing 1500 kgm on the cycle ergometer (see figure 4.17). This test became known as the PWC 170 (physical working capacity at a heart rate of 170) test, and it was used to predict the amount of work an individual would perform if that individual were to cycle up to a heart rate of 170 beats/min.

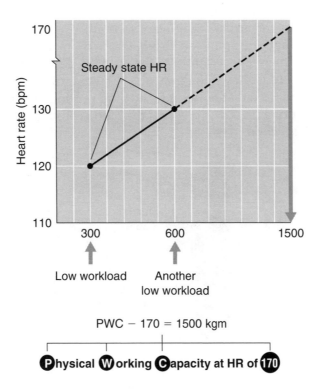

Figure 4.17 The PWC 170 test.

Another researcher working with female swimmers modified the test to a PWC 150, the amount of work the study subjects would be doing if they were to work to a heart rate of 150 beats/min. Thus the workload for any heart rate can be predicted from the relationship between heart rate and workload. The YMCA, when it developed its test, decided to use PWC max, which predicts how much work a subject would be doing if that individual were working at his or her maximum heart rate. Remember that maximum heart rate is determined by the 220 – age formula.

Blood

Blood is the fluid that moves through the circulatory system. We have all seen it, felt it, and may have even tasted it. Blood is more viscous than water, partially because blood is the main transportation system of the body. Many solids are in the blood because anything that is going from one place in the body to another gets there through the bloodstream.

Blood consists of red blood cells, white blood cells, and blood platelets. Blood also contains the hundreds of substances that it is transporting in the body. All the nutrients (carbohydrates, fats, amino acids, etc.) in their component forms are being transported in the blood and can be measured. Respiratory gases must travel in the bloodstream to be delivered to the muscles or the lungs. All the waste products, the end products of muscle metabolism and protein breakdown, represent a large group of substances being transported that can be found in the blood. In addition, other substances like blood enzymes, antigens and antibodies, and hormones from the endocrine glands can be found in the blood.

If a test tube (regardless of its size) were filled with whole blood and then put into a centrifuge and spun at a high rate, the more dense substances in the blood would be thrown to the bottom of the centrifuge tube. After spinning, the blood would separate as shown in figure 4.18. The top part is *serum* (or plasma), a light straw-colored fluid that represents the fluid portion of the blood. The lower part, which is a very dark red, represents the blood cells and other solids in the blood. It is called *hematocrit*.

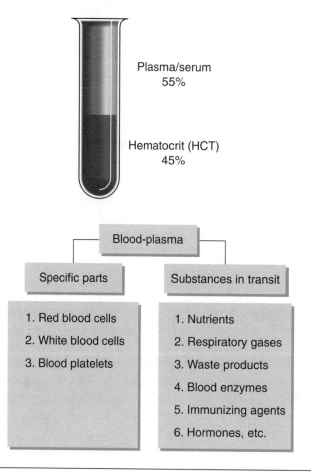

Figure 4.18 Components of blood.

The division is almost half and half, with just a little more serum present (55% of the sample) than the hematocrit (45% of the sample). If you were to jog on a hot day and became dehydrated, then took a sample of blood and centrifuged it, the serum might now be 45% and the hematocrit 55% (just the opposite). During dehydration, fluid from the plasma is lost. This test is a very simple way to determine if an individual is dehydrated.

Figure 4.18 further classifies the blood into two categories: specific parts and substances in transit. The specific parts of the blood are the blood cells, and the substances in transit comprise all the substances the blood is transporting throughout the body. As noted earlier, the blood is the transportation system of the body. A good physiology textbook will list under "composition of blood" all the substances in the blood and the normal amounts of each substance, as well as what it means if the amount is higher or lower than normal. To make it easier to understand, we have grouped these substances into large categories as shown in figure 4.18. Nutrients, for example, consist of hundreds of substances: all the sugars and carbohydrates; all the amino acids; all the fatty acids, vitamins, and minerals; and so on.

All the substances that the blood transports have normal values. These values are often reported as how much of that substance is in 100 milliliters (ml) of blood. Here are some common examples. Cholesterol has become a household term and has been linked to coronary heart disease. The American Heart Association would like all adults to have a total cholesterol level of less than 200 milligrams (mg) per 100 ml of blood (or 200mg/100 ml). Sometimes this formula is written as 200mg/dl; a dl is a *deciliter* or one 10th of a liter, which is again 100 ml. Or it might be reported as 200 mg%; again, percent is per 100. Other common examples are normal levels of triglycerides, which are 50 to 150 mg per 100 ml of blood, and of glucose, which are 80 to 100 mg per 100 ml of blood.

We turn now to a discussion of hemoglobin. Hemoglobin is found in the red blood cell and is responsible for transporting oxygen. Hemoglobin (hb) is made up of protein, pigment, and iron and has a great affinity for oxygen. It carries oxygen in the blood in a loose chemical combination. As with other substances in the blood, it is common to express hemoglobin values by how much hemoglobin is in 100 ml of blood. Normally 14 to 16 grams (g) of hemoglobin are found per 100 ml of blood. As we know that 1 g of hemoglobin can carry 1.34 ml of oxygen, we can calculate with simple arithmetic how much oxygen will be in 100 ml of blood. At the low end of the scale, if there were 14 g of hb per 100 ml of blood and each gram carried 1.34 ml of oxygen, then there would be 18.76 ml of oxygen per 100 ml of blood ($14 \times 1.34 = 18.76$). However, if there were 15 g of hb/100 ml, then the amount of oxygen in 100 ml of blood would be 20.1 ml ($15 \times 1.34 = 20.1$). If the hemoglobin were at the top of the range and had 16 g of hb per 100 ml of blood, then 100 ml of blood would carry 21.44 ml of oxygen ($16 \times 1.34 = 21.44$). If there were 14.7 g of hb per 100 ml of blood, then 100 ml of blood would carry 19.7 ml of oxygen ($14.7 \times 1.34 = 19.7$). So the amount of oxygen carried by 100 ml of blood depends, in part, on the amount of hemoglobin in the blood.

Textbooks usually round these numbers off to 20 ml per 100 ml of blood, but instead of calling it 20 ml/100 ml of blood textbooks will refer to 20 vpc. The abbreviation *vpc* is volumes percent or milliliters per 100 milliliters. So the oxygen-carrying capacity of blood is said to be 20 vpc. Depending on the amount of hemoglobin present, the 20 vpc estimate may or may not be correct; however, 20 vpc is a good generalization.

When the hemoglobin is carrying all the oxygen possible (i.e., every gram of hemoglobin is carrying 1.34 ml of oxygen), the blood is said to be *fully saturated*; that is, it cannot carry any more oxygen. Arterial blood is fully saturated. Venous blood, in contrast, gives up some of its oxygen when it passes through the muscle capillaries and therefore is not fully saturated but is something less. How much less depends on how much oxygen was given to the tissues.

Although the blood seldom becomes 100% saturated due to partial pressures of gases, let's assume for the sake of simplicity that fully saturated is 100% saturated. We could say that arterial blood is fully saturated or has 20 vpc of oxygen in it and that venous blood is less than fully saturated. Using 100% as fully saturated, if 100 ml of blood gave up 10 vpc of oxygen as it passed through the muscle tissue, the venous blood would be 50% saturated (there would be 10 vpc of oxygen in it). If 20 vpc is 100% saturated, then 10 vpc is 50% saturated, 5 vpc is 25%

saturated, and so on. By simple arithmetic we can determine how much oxygen the blood is carrying. Arterial blood carries 20 ml per 100 ml of blood (20 vpc). If venous blood is 68% saturated, then the venous blood is carrying 13.6 vpc (68% of 20 vpc). If the blood is 79% saturated, then the blood is carrying 15.8 vpc of oxygen (0.79 × 20).

These examples also explain another term, *AVO₂ difference*, which is the difference between the amount of oxygen in the arterial blood and the amount of oxygen in the venous blood. If the arterial blood is carrying 20 vpc of oxygen and the venous blood is carrying 11 vpc of oxygen, this means that every 100 ml of blood that passed through the muscle gave up 9 vpc of oxygen. This is the AVO_2 difference (arterial blood 20 vpc minus venous blood 11 vpc = AVO_2 difference of 9 vpc). In this example each 100 ml of blood gave up 9 ml of oxygen.

At this point let's review three terms:

■ Heart rate (HR) is the number of times the heart beats (or pumps) per minute.

■ Stroke volume (SV) is how much blood the heart pumps on each contraction.

■ Cardiac output (Q) is the amount of blood pumped by the heart in a minute, or minute volume. Cardiac output is the product of heart rate and stroke volume ($HR \times SV = Q$).

Therefore, if the volume of blood being pumped is known (Q), you should be able to determine how much oxygen that much blood is transporting. An example will illustrate. If the heart rate (HR) is 70 beats/min and the stroke volume (SV) is 80 ml, then the cardiac output is 5600 ml ($70 \times 80 = 5600$ ml) or 5.6 liters per minute ($L \cdot min^{-1}$) (1000 ml = 1 L). If 20% of the blood is oxygen (20 ml/100 ml), then 5.6 liters of blood is transporting 1.12 liters of oxygen per minute ($0.2 \times 5.6 = 1.12$). This formula does not mean that the body *needs* 1.12 liters of oxygen per minute; it just means that the blood is transporting 1.12 liters of blood per minute. When that blood passes through the muscle it gives up some of its oxygen and the amount of oxygen given to the muscle depends on how much O_2 is needed. When the venous blood is returned to the lungs, the amount of oxygen that was unloaded must be picked up in the lungs to bring the blood back up to full saturation. This amount is called the oxygen uptake ($\dot{V}O_2$).

Oxygen uptake is the amount of oxygen that is picked up by the blood in the lungs in one minute. In its simplest form, oxygen uptake is the amount of oxygen exhaled subtracted from the amount of oxygen inhaled, expressed per minute ($VIO_2 - VEO_2 = \dot{V}O_2$). VIO_2 is the inspired oxygen and VEO_2 is the expired oxygen. The volume of air breathed in has to be measured and the amount of oxygen in that inspired air calculated. Likewise the air breathed out has to be analyzed to determine the oxygen content. Expressed per minute, the difference is oxygen uptake. If it's measured while the subject is at rest, it's called the *resting oxygen uptake*; if it's measured while the subject is doing any kind of work, at any intensity, it's called *exercise oxygen uptake*. Last, if it's measured while the subject is doing a maximum task, it's called the *maximum oxygen uptake*.

How much oxygen a person takes up at rest depends on the person's size. A 200-pound man needs more oxygen than a 100-pound woman. He has a larger muscle mass, larger bones, larger viscera, a larger heart, and larger lungs, and therefore he needs more oxygen than the woman doing the same thing.

Before we continue with oxygen uptake, let's do a short review of the respiratory system. We are talking about oxygen transportation, but where does the oxygen come from? The air. And how does the oxygen in the air get into the blood? Through the respiratory system. The circulatory and respiratory systems are intimately involved in the transportation of oxygen.

Respiratory System

The definition of respiration is the exchange of oxygen and carbon dioxide. This definition is the case regardless of whether one is talking about plants or animals. Humans have three kinds of respiration: external, internal, and cellular.

- *External respiration* is the exchange of oxygen and carbon dioxide between the air in the environment and the air in the lungs.

- *Internal respiration* is the exchange of oxygen and carbon dioxide between the air in the lungs and the blood in the lungs. Remember pulmonary circulation? All the blood of the body goes from the heart to the lungs and back to the heart. Also the air we breathe in goes into the lungs. Although the air and blood do not mix mechanically, the blood in the thin-walled capillaries and the air in the thin-walled alveoli enable the O_2 and the CO_2 to pass through the capillary walls, making the exchange.

- *Cellular respiration* is the exchange of oxygen and carbon dioxide between the blood in the capillaries and the muscle cells.

If an individual is connected to a spirometer, his or her breathing pattern can be drawn on a graph. Terms can be assigned to the different volumes of air. Figure 4.19 shows the breathing pattern for an average adult at rest.

Here are the terms that you should know, with their definitions:

- *Tidal volume* (TV) is the amount of air that is taken in and out with each breath. In the average adult at rest this is 500 ml.

- *Inspiratory reserve volume* (IRV) is the maximum amount of air that can be inspired after a normal inspiration. In the average adult at rest this is 3000 ml (3 L).

- *Expiratory reserve volume* (ERV) is the maximum amount of air that can be exhaled after a normal expiration. In the average adult at rest it is about one-third of the IRV or 1000 ml.

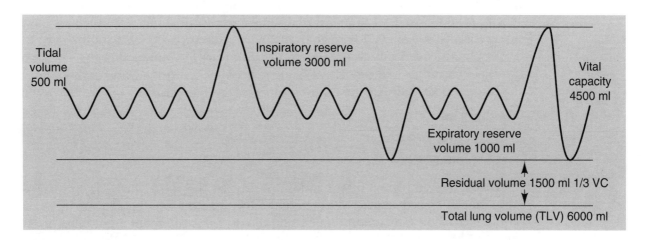

Figure 4.19 Lung volume patterns for adults.

- *Vital capacity* is the sum of TV, IRV, and ERV, or the maximum amount of air that can be inhaled and exhaled. In the average adult this is 4500 ml (4.5 L).
- *Residual volume* (RV) is the volume of air that remains in the lungs after a maximal expiration. The air passageways (trachea, bronchi, and bronchioles) have noncollapsible walls, so even after a full expiration the air in those airways cannot be expelled. This situation is sometimes called dead air in dead air spaces. In the average adult this is about one-third of the vital capacity or 1500 ml.
- *Total lung volume* (TLV) is the vital capacity added to the residual volume. In the average adult this volume is 6000 ml (6 L).

When a person exercises, the terms and definitions of these volumes remain the same, but the numerical values differ depending on how hard the person is working (see figure 4.20).

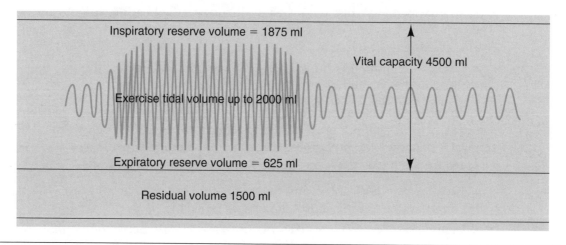

Figure 4.20 Exercising values for lung volumes.

Each definition is exactly the same, but the sizes of the volumes have changed. Tidal volume is still the amount of air taken in with each breath, except now this is a very large volume because an exercising individual is breathing deeply and fast. The other volumes must necessarily change because more of the vital capacity is being used for tidal volume. Vital capacity, residual volume, and total lung volume, however, do not change during exercise.

We breathe primarily to obtain oxygen from the air. Atmospheric air is a remarkably accurate and consistent mixture of oxygen, nitrogen, and carbon dioxide. Atmospheric air has the following percentages of gases:

- Oxygen = 20.93%
- Nitrogen = 79%
- Carbon dioxide = 0.04%

Nitrogen is simply a dilutant and is not used by the body. The body's metabolism, however, is designed to exist on a reduced mixture of oxygen. Because air contains such a small amount of carbon dioxide, it is often not mentioned as an element of air, and the composition of air is simply given as 20% oxygen and 80% nitrogen. (Using these imprecise percentages is not applicable to research or advanced work, but, for our purposes, they are easy to remember and to use in mental arithmetic.)

Some review of definitions is in order:

- *Respiration rate* (RR and sometimes *f* for *frequency*) is how many times a person breathes in one minute. In humans RR at rest covers a large range, from 10 to 20 times a minute. The average is 15 times a minute.
- *Tidal volume* (TV) is the amount of air taken in with each breath, which is 500 ml at rest.
- *Minute volume* ($\dot{V}E$) is the amount of air breathed in a minute. $\dot{V}E$ stands for volume expired in a minute. It could have been called $\dot{V}I$ (the volume inspired in a minute) but it is always measured from expired air, hence the acronym $\dot{V}E$. $\dot{V}E$ is the product of respiration rate (RR) and tidal volume (TV). Using the above figures to calculate the $\dot{V}E$ for an adult at rest, we arrive at the figure of 7500 ml ($15 \times 500 = 7500$).

In this example of a $\dot{V}E$ of 7500 ml, the 7500 ml is the amount of atmospheric air inspired in a minute. If 20% of the air is oxygen, 1500 ml of oxygen will be present in that amount of air ($0.2 \times 7500 = 1500$) or 1500 ml of oxygen per minute. Actually we only require a small amount of the oxygen, so the oxygen we do not use is exhaled. If we take the inspired oxygen (1500 ml) and subtract the expired oxygen (this has to be measured with a gas analyzer) and assume that for this example there were 1300 ml of oxygen in the expired air, the difference is 200 ml. Two hundred millileters is the *oxygen uptake* ($\dot{V}O_2$).

Putting the concepts and figures just described into an arithmetic model helps to illustrate the relationship between all the circulatory and respiratory terms (see figure 4.21).

Figure 4.21 is only a model and contains some assumptions and errors that will be explained at the end of this section. Following is an explanation of the model presented in figure 4.21.

- Column 1 lists what the subject is doing. First the subject is at rest; then the subject is working on a cycle ergometer with increasing workloads until he or she cannot continue.

Condition	HR (bpm)	SV (ml)	$\dot{Q}$ (L)	Amount O_2 in $\dot{Q}$	Amount O_2 needed	Amount O_2 unloaded	Respiration rate	TV (ml)	$\dot{V}E$ (L)	Amount O_2 in $\dot{V}E$	$\dot{V}O_2$ (L)
Rest	70	80	5.6	1.12	0.2	0.2	15	500	7.5	1.5	0.2
300kgm	110	95	10.45	2.09	1.3	1.3	35	1200	42	8.4	1.3
600kgm	136	110	14.96	2.99	2.4	2.4	45	1400	63	12.6	2.4
900kgm	162	120	19.44	3.89	3.5	3.5	60	1500	90	18	3.5
1200kgm	190	120	22.8	4.56	4.56	4.56	80	1700	136	27.2	4.56
1350kgm	190	120	22.8	4.56	5.2	4.56	90	1850	166	33.2	4.56

Figure 4.21 $\dot{V}O_2$ arithmetic model.

▪ Column 2 is the subject's heart rate, first at rest and then increasing as the workload increases. Once the subject's workload reaches 1200 kgm, even an increase in workload does not increase the heart rate, and 190 beats/min is therefore the subject's maximum heart rate.

▪ Column 3 is the subject's stroke volume. At rest we are assuming that this subject had a stroke volume of 80 ml, which is an average stroke volume for an unconditioned average person. During exercise blood pressure increases, and therefore the stroke volume increases as well. The heart fills during the time between two heartbeats (diastole), and when the blood pressure is higher, more blood is pushed into the heart during that time. Stroke volume continues to increase up to about 60% of the subject's maximum capacity and then levels off. This leveling off occurs because even though the blood pressure continues to rise, the time between two beats is so short that the heart does not have a chance to inject more blood.

▪ Column 4 is cardiac output and is the product of HR × SV. Cardiac output is the amount of blood being pumped per minute and is given in liters.

▪ Column 5 is an academic or informational column and simply gives the amount of oxygen that is being transported in that amount of blood. (20% of blood is oxygen.)

▪ Column 6 is the amount of oxygen needed for that particular workload. These figures have been estimated based on the observation that the amount of oxygen needed is a function of size. At rest an average woman (57 kg) will need about 200 ml or 0.2 L of oxygen per minute. As the subject increases the workload, the amount of oxygen needed is increased.

▪ Column 7 is the actual amount of oxygen that is given up to the tissue. The blood is carrying much more oxygen than is needed (see column 5), so that usually the amount of oxygen unloaded is the amount the muscles need.

▪ Column 8 is the respiration rate. At rest it is 15 breaths per minute, but as the subject works harder the rate of respiration increases.

▪ Column 9 is the depth of each breath or tidal volume (TV), starting at rest with a tidal volume of 500 ml and increasing as the workload increases.

▪ Column 10 is the minute volume ($\dot{V}E$) and is the product of respiration rate and tidal volume. $\dot{V}E$ is the amount of air being breathed in and out of the lungs in one minute and is given in liters.

▪ Column 11 is again an academic or informational column calculating how much oxygen is in the air breathed in and out (20% of $\dot{V}E$).

▪ Column 12 is the oxygen uptake ($\dot{V}O_2$); that is, of the oxygen breathed in, the amount of oxygen actually picked up by the blood to once again bring the blood to full saturation. For example, at rest the amount of oxygen in the $\dot{V}E$ was 1.5 liters (20% of 7.5 liters). However, the subject needed only 0.2 liters of the 1.5 liters, because only 0.2 liters was unloaded at the tissue level. The amount of oxygen needed to again saturate the blood is the same as the amount that was unloaded. At a workload of 600 kgm the $\dot{V}E$ was 63 liters per minute ($L \cdot min^{-1}$), of which 12.6 liters were oxygen, but at a workload of 300 kgm (or workload 1) the subject needed only 1.3 liters of oxygen to replace that which was unloaded at the tissue level. At a workload of 1200 kgm, the model shows that all the oxygen the blood was carrying was unloaded (4.56 L), so in the lungs the $\dot{V}E$ was

136 liters and contained 27.2 liters of oxygen, but the blood picked up only 4.56 liters of oxygen. This is because the 22.8 liters of blood (Q at that workload) can carry only 4.56 liters of oxygen. At the final workload of 1350 kgm the cardiac output did not increase, so the amount of blood delivered is the same amount of oxygen as during the previous workload. The subject is working harder and needs more oxygen, but the blood cannot unload more than it's carrying, so the muscles have to work without oxygen (anaerobically). In the lungs the blood can still pick up only 4.56 liters of oxygen because that's all 22.8 liters of blood can carry, and maximum oxygen uptake has been attained.

Figure 4.21 is only a model, and although the model is technically correct, it does contain some errors. The model does illustrate, however, how all these functions work together to deliver oxygen to the working muscles. For example, it appears in the model that anaerobic work (work without oxygen) started at the last workload. The subject needed 5.2 liters of oxygen but the blood could only supply 4.56 liters. In reality, anaerobic work started much earlier, probably in the second workload. This error in the model occurs because the model is assuming that all of the blood ($\dot{Q}$) is going to where it is needed. Much of the blood ($\dot{Q}$) goes to parts of the body that do not require much more oxygen (brain, viscera, liver, bones, etc.) during exercise. In column 6 it is assumed that all the blood is going to the working muscles, so that the numbers in this column are inflated.

It can also be noted that in the lungs there is no shortage of oxygen. At every workload more oxygen is being breathed in than can possibly be used. It isn't the lungs that can't supply the oxygen, but the inability of the blood to transport it from the lungs to the tissue. During the final workload, when the subject reached maximum workload and maximum oxygen uptake, 33.2 liters of oxygen were available in the lungs, but the blood could only pick up and carry 4.56 liters.

Measurement of Oxygen Uptake

Oxygen uptake ($\dot{V}O_2$) is measured for several reasons. Maximum oxygen uptake, or $\dot{V}O_2max$, is considered to be one of the best measures of aerobic fitness. The more oxygen that can be delivered to the muscle tissue, the more work the muscles can do. If physiologists were asked to test an athlete's fitness but were restricted to using only one test, most would choose $\dot{V}O_2max$. The maximum oxygen uptake is an excellent test of cardiorespiratory efficiency and is often mentioned in both scientific and popular literature.

The measurement of $\dot{V}O_2max$ is a laboratory technique that involves both the collection and the analysis of expired air during exercise; however, as it is known that both heart rate and oxygen uptake have a linear relationship to workload, it is possible to predict the maximum oxygen uptake from heart rate values. As the workload increases, the heart rate and the oxygen uptake also increase. This relationship allows the prediction of a maximum oxygen uptake from the maximum heart rate.

Two other reasons $\dot{V}O_2$ is measured, which are discussed in greater detail in later sections of this chapter, are to determine the caloric cost of exercise and to measure activity intensity. Before looking at the other uses of measuring $\dot{V}O_2$, we explain how oxygen uptakes can be equalized among people of different weights to allow their uptakes to be compared.

Equalizing Oxygen Uptake

The amount of oxygen needed for any task is a function of size (i.e., weight), so oxygen uptakes among individuals only can be compared if weight is equalized among participants, including males and females. Figure 4.22 illustrates a man and a woman climbing a flight of stairs together. The man weighs 200 pounds (90.9 kg) and the female weighs 100 pounds (45.5 kg). They are climbing the same stairs at the same speed, so they are doing the same task. However, the man is carrying twice the weight of the woman, so it's reasonable to assume that he is doing twice as much work as the woman.

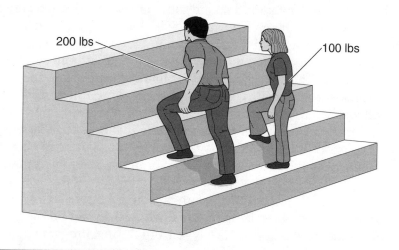

200 lbs   100 lbs

Figure 4.22   Weight as a factor in oxygen uptake.

It is easy to express work when stepping by using a formula to determine the number of units known as foot per pounds of work.

Work (in ft lb/min) = Distance × Resistance × Speed

Assume that the height of the step is 12 inches and the speed of climbing the stairs is 24 steps per minute. Insert these figures into the formula to determine the work accomplished by the man and woman climbing the steps:

Distance = 12 in. (the height of the step)

Resistance = 200 lbs for the man and 100 lbs for the woman (body weight)

Speed = 24 steps per minute (the speed of stepping)

As the formula is for foot pounds, change the height of the step into feet (12 in. = 1 ft).

For the man: 1 × 200 × 24 = 4800 foot pounds per minute

For the woman: 1 × 100 × 24 = 2400 foot pounds per minute

The man is doing twice as much work as the woman because he weighs twice as much she does. It is also reasonable to assume that if he is doing twice as much work, he needs twice as much oxygen. Only body weight makes the difference. If the oxygen uptake were actually measured, the oxygen uptake would be as follows:

$$\text{For the man: } \dot{V}O_2 = 1.273 \text{ L} \cdot \text{min}^{-1}$$

$$\text{For the woman: } \dot{V}O_2 = 0.637 \text{ L} \cdot \text{min}^{-1}$$

For us to compare their work, the man and woman in our example must weigh the same. Weight must be factored out. We factor out the weight by dividing the oxygen uptake by body weight and expressing the oxygen uptake per unit of body weight. As the numbers will be less than one liter, it is easier to change the $\dot{V}O_2$ into milliliters and then divide by their body weight in kilograms, expressing the $\dot{V}O_2$ per kilogram of body weight as follows:

For the man: $\dot{V}O_2 = 1.273 \text{ L} = 1273 \text{ ml/min}$, divided by 90.9 kg (200 lbs) $= 14 \text{ ml} \cdot \text{kg}^{-1} \cdot \text{min}^{-1}$

For the woman: $\dot{V}O_2 = 0.637 \text{ L} = 637 \text{ ml/min}$, divided by 45.5 kg (100 lbs) $= 14 \text{ ml} \cdot \text{kg}^{-1} \cdot \text{min}^{-1}$

When individuals weigh the same and do the same task, they use the same amount of oxygen. Figure 4.23 illustrates the man and woman climbing the stairs, and their weight has been divided into one-kilogram blocks.

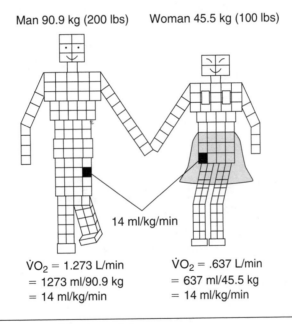

Man 90.9 kg (200 lbs)   Woman 45.5 kg (100 lbs)

14 ml/kg/min

$\dot{V}O_2 = 1.273 \text{ L/min}$
$= 1273 \text{ ml/90.9 kg}$
$= 14 \text{ ml/kg/min}$

$\dot{V}O_2 = .637 \text{ L/min}$
$= 637 \text{ ml/45.5 kg}$
$= 14 \text{ ml/kg/min}$

Figure 4.23 $\dot{V}O_2$ per kilogram of body weight.

To compare any individuals, male to male or male to female, $\dot{V}O_2$ must be expressed per kilogram of body weight. Expressing the weight in this fashion equalizes the subjects' weights so comparisons can be made. This is accomplished by dividing the oxygen uptake by the body weight. (*Note*: For ease of calculation, convert oxygen uptake from liters per minute to milliliters per minute by multiplying by 1000; then divide by body weight in kilograms. This conversion will give the oxygen in milliliters per kilogram [ml/kg]. Because oxygen uptake is always given per minute, this expression becomes ml/kg/min, or $\text{ml} \cdot \text{kg}^{-1} \cdot \text{min}^{-1}$. Table 4.1 gives all $\dot{V}O_2$ in L and ml/kg.)

Table 4.1 Maximum Oxygen Uptake Conversion Chart (L/kg/min to ml/kg/min)

Body weight		Maximum oxygen uptake (L/kg/min)																																												
lb	kg	1.5	1.6	1.7	1.8	1.9	2.0	2.1	2.2	2.3	2.4	2.5	2.6	2.7	2.8	2.9	3.0	3.1	3.2	3.3	3.4	3.5	3.6	3.7	3.8	3.9	4.0	4.1	4.2	4.3	4.4	4.5	4.6	4.7	4.8	4.9	5.0	5.1	5.2	5.3	5.4	5.5	5.6	5.7	5.8	5.9	6.0
110	50	30	32	34	36	38	40	42	44	46	48	50	52	54	56	58	60	62	64	66	68	70	72	74	76	78	80	82	84	86	88	90	92	94	96	98	100	102	104	106	108	110	112	114	116	118	120
112	51	29	31	33	35	37	39	41	43	45	47	49	51	53	55	57	59	61	63	65	67	69	71	73	75	76	78	80	82	84	86	88	90	92	94	96	98	100	102	104	106	108	110	112	114	116	118
115	52	29	31	33	35	37	38	40	42	44	46	48	50	52	54	56	58	60	62	63	65	67	69	71	73	75	77	79	81	83	85	87	88	90	92	94	96	98	100	102	104	106	108	110	112	113	115
117	53	28	30	32	34	36	38	40	42	43	45	47	49	51	53	55	57	58	60	62	64	66	68	70	72	74	75	77	79	81	83	85	87	89	91	92	94	96	98	100	102	104	106	108	109	111	113
119	54	28	30	31	33	35	37	39	41	43	44	46	48	50	52	54	56	57	59	61	63	65	67	69	70	72	74	76	78	80	81	83	85	87	89	91	93	94	96	98	100	102	104	106	107	109	111
121	55	27	29	31	33	35	36	38	40	42	44	45	47	49	51	53	55	56	58	60	62	64	65	67	69	71	73	75	76	78	80	82	84	85	87	89	91	93	95	96	98	100	102	104	105	107	109
123	56	27	29	30	32	34	36	38	39	41	43	45	46	48	50	52	54	55	57	59	61	63	64	66	68	70	71	73	75	77	79	80	82	84	86	88	89	91	93	95	96	98	100	102	104	105	107
126	57	26	28	30	32	33	35	37	39	40	42	44	46	47	49	51	53	54	56	58	60	61	63	65	67	68	70	72	74	75	77	79	81	82	84	86	88	89	91	93	95	96	98	100	102	104	105
128	58	26	28	29	31	33	34	36	38	40	41	43	45	47	48	50	52	53	55	57	59	60	62	64	66	67	69	71	72	74	76	78	79	81	83	84	86	88	90	91	93	95	97	98	100	102	103
130	59	25	27	29	31	32	34	36	37	39	41	42	44	46	47	49	51	53	54	56	58	59	61	63	64	66	68	69	71	73	75	76	78	80	81	83	85	86	88	90	92	93	95	97	98	100	102
132	60	25	27	28	30	32	33	35	37	38	40	42	43	45	47	48	50	52	53	55	57	58	60	62	63	65	67	68	70	72	73	75	77	78	80	82	83	85	87	88	90	92	93	95	97	98	100
134	61	25	26	28	30	31	33	34	36	38	39	41	43	44	46	48	49	51	52	54	56	57	59	61	62	64	66	67	69	70	72	74	75	77	79	80	82	84	85	87	89	90	92	93	95	97	98
137	62	24	26	27	29	31	32	34	35	37	39	40	42	44	45	47	48	50	52	53	55	56	58	60	61	63	65	66	68	69	71	73	74	76	77	79	81	82	84	85	87	89	90	92	94	95	97
139	63	24	25	27	29	30	32	33	35	37	38	40	41	43	44	46	48	49	51	52	54	56	57	59	60	62	63	65	67	68	70	71	73	75	76	78	79	81	83	84	86	87	89	90	92	94	95
141	64	23	25	27	28	30	31	33	34	36	38	39	41	42	44	45	47	48	50	52	53	55	56	58	59	61	63	64	66	67	69	70	72	73	75	77	78	80	81	83	84	86	88	89	91	92	94
143	65	23	25	26	28	29	31	32	34	35	37	38	40	42	43	45	46	48	49	51	52	54	55	57	58	60	62	63	65	66	68	69	71	72	74	75	77	78	80	82	83	85	86	88	89	91	92
146	66	23	24	26	27	29	30	32	33	35	36	38	39	41	42	44	45	47	48	50	52	53	55	56	58	59	61	62	64	65	67	68	70	71	73	74	76	77	79	80	82	83	85	86	88	89	91
148	67	22	24	25	27	28	30	31	33	34	36	37	39	40	42	43	45	46	48	49	51	52	54	55	57	58	60	61	63	64	66	67	69	70	72	73	75	76	78	79	81	82	84	85	87	88	90
150	68	22	24	25	26	28	29	31	32	34	35	37	38	40	41	43	44	46	47	49	50	51	53	54	56	57	59	60	62	63	65	66	68	69	71	72	74	75	76	78	79	81	82	84	85	87	88
152	69	22	23	25	26	28	29	30	32	33	35	36	38	39	41	42	43	45	46	48	49	51	52	54	55	57	58	59	61	62	64	65	67	68	70	71	72	74	75	77	78	80	81	83	84	86	87
154	70	21	23	24	26	27	29	30	31	33	34	36	37	39	40	41	43	44	46	47	49	50	51	53	54	56	57	59	60	61	63	64	66	67	69	70	71	73	74	76	77	79	80	81	83	84	86
157	71	21	23	24	25	27	28	30	31	32	34	35	37	38	39	41	42	44	45	46	48	49	51	52	54	55	56	58	59	61	62	63	65	66	68	69	70	72	73	75	76	77	79	80	82	83	85
159	72	21	22	24	25	26	28	29	31	32	33	35	36	38	39	40	42	43	44	46	47	49	50	51	53	54	56	57	58	60	61	63	64	65	67	68	69	71	72	74	75	76	78	79	81	82	83
161	73	21	22	23	25	26	27	29	30	32	33	34	36	37	38	40	41	42	44	45	47	48	49	51	52	53	55	56	58	59	60	62	63	64	66	67	68	70	71	73	74	75	77	78	79	81	82
163	74	20	22	23	24	26	27	28	30	31	32	34	35	36	38	39	41	42	43	45	46	47	49	50	51	53	54	55	57	58	59	61	62	64	65	66	68	69	70	72	73	74	76	77	78	80	81
165	75	20	21	23	24	25	27	28	29	31	32	33	35	36	37	39	40	41	43	44	45	47	48	49	51	52	53	55	56	57	59	60	61	63	64	65	67	68	69	71	72	73	75	76	77	79	80
168	76	20	21	22	24	25	26	28	29	30	32	33	34	36	37	38	39	41	42	43	45	46	47	49	50	51	53	54	55	57	58	59	61	62	63	64	66	67	68	70	71	72	74	75	76	78	79
170	77	19	21	22	23	25	26	27	29	30	31	32	34	35	36	38	39	40	42	43	44	45	47	48	49	51	52	53	55	56	57	58	60	61	62	64	65	66	68	69	70	71	73	74	75	77	78
172	78	19	21	22	23	24	26	27	28	29	31	32	33	35	36	37	38	40	41	42	44	45	46	47	49	50	51	53	54	55	56	58	59	60	62	63	64	65	67	68	69	71	72	73	74	76	77
174	79	19	20	22	23	24	25	27	28	29	30	32	33	34	35	37	38	39	41	42	43	44	46	47	48	49	51	52	53	54	56	57	58	59	61	62	63	65	66	67	68	70	71	72	73	75	76
176	80	19	20	21	23	24	25	26	28	29	30	31	33	34	35	36	38	39	40	41	43	44	45	46	48	49	50	51	53	54	55	56	58	59	60	61	63	64	65	66	68	69	70	71	73	74	75
179	81	19	20	21	22	23	25	26	27	28	30	31	32	33	35	36	37	38	40	41	42	43	44	46	47	48	49	51	52	53	54	56	57	58	59	60	62	63	64	65	67	68	69	70	72	73	74
181	82	18	20	21	22	23	24	26	27	28	29	30	32	33	34	35	37	38	39	40	41	43	44	45	46	48	49	50	51	52	54	55	56	57	59	60	61	62	63	65	66	67	68	70	71	72	73
183	83	18	19	20	22	23	24	25	27	28	29	30	31	33	34	35	36	37	39	40	41	42	43	45	46	47	48	49	51	52	53	54	55	57	58	59	60	61	63	64	65	66	67	69	70	71	72
185	84	18	19	20	21	23	24	25	26	27	29	30	31	32	33	35	36	37	38	39	40	42	43	44	45	46	48	49	50	51	52	54	55	56	57	58	60	61	62	63	64	65	67	68	69	70	71
187	85	18	19	20	21	22	24	25	26	27	28	29	31	32	33	34	35	36	38	39	40	41	42	44	45	46	47	48	49	51	52	53	54	55	56	58	59	60	61	62	64	65	66	67	68	69	71
190	86	17	19	20	21	22	23	24	26	27	28	29	30	31	33	34	35	36	37	38	40	41	42	43	44	45	47	48	49	50	51	52	53	55	56	57	58	59	60	62	63	64	65	66	67	69	70
192	87	17	18	20	21	22	23	24	25	26	28	29	30	31	32	33	34	36	37	38	39	40	41	43	44	45	46	47	48	49	51	52	53	54	55	56	57	59	60	61	62	63	64	66	67	68	69
194	88	17	18	19	20	22	23	24	25	26	27	28	30	31	32	33	34	35	36	38	39	40	41	42	43	44	45	47	48	49	50	51	52	53	55	56	57	58	59	60	61	63	64	65	66	67	68
196	89	17	18	19	20	21	22	24	25	26	27	28	29	30	31	33	34	35	36	37	38	39	40	42	43	44	45	46	47	48	49	51	52	53	54	55	56	57	58	60	61	62	63	64	65	66	67
198	90	17	18	19	20	21	22	23	24	26	27	28	29	30	31	32	33	34	36	37	38	39	40	41	42	43	44	46	47	48	49	50	51	52	53	54	56	57	58	59	60	61	62	63	64	66	67
201	91	16	18	19	20	21	22	23	24	25	26	27	29	30	31	32	33	34	35	36	37	38	40	41	42	43	44	45	46	47	48	49	51	52	53	54	55	56	57	58	59	60	62	63	64	65	66
203	92	16	17	18	20	21	22	23	24	25	26	27	28	29	30	32	33	34	35	36	37	38	39	40	41	42	43	45	46	47	48	49	50	51	52	53	54	55	57	58	59	60	61	62	63	64	65
205	93	16	17	18	19	20	22	23	24	25	26	27	28	29	30	31	32	33	34	35	37	38	39	40	41	42	43	44	45	46	47	48	49	51	52	53	54	55	56	57	58	59	60	61	62	63	65
207	94	16	17	18	19	20	21	22	23	24	26	27	28	29	30	31	32	33	34	35	36	37	38	39	40	41	43	44	45	46	47	48	49	50	51	52	53	54	55	56	57	59	60	61	62	63	64
209	95	16	17	18	19	20	21	22	23	24	25	26	27	28	29	31	32	33	34	35	36	37	38	39	40	41	42	43	44	45	46	47	48	49	51	52	53	54	55	56	57	58	59	60	61	62	63
212	96	16	17	18	19	20	21	22	23	24	25	26	27	28	29	30	31	32	33	34	35	36	38	39	40	41	42	43	44	45	46	47	48	49	50	51	52	53	54	55	56	57	58	59	60	61	63
214	97	15	16	18	19	20	21	22	23	24	25	26	27	28	29	30	31	32	33	34	35	36	37	38	39	40	41	42	43	44	45	46	47	48	49	51	52	53	54	55	56	57	58	59	60	61	62
216	98	15	16	17	18	19	20	21	22	23	24	26	27	28	29	30	31	32	33	34	35	36	37	38	39	40	41	42	43	44	45	46	47	48	49	50	51	52	53	54	55	56	57	58	59	60	61
218	99	15	16	17	18	19	20	21	22	23	24	25	26	27	28	29	30	31	32	33	34	35	36	37	38	39	40	41	42	43	44	45	46	47	48	49	51	52	53	54	55	56	57	58	59	60	61
220	100	15	16	17	18	19	20	21	22	23	24	25	26	27	28	29	30	31	32	33	34	35	36	37	38	39	40	41	42	43	44	45	46	47	48	49	50	51	52	53	54	55	56	57	58	59	60

Reprinted by permission from Work Tests With the Bicycle Ergometer (p. 14) by P.-O. Åstrand, n.d., Varberg, Sweden: Monark. Copyright by Monark AB.

Caloric Cost of Exercise

Oxygen uptake is also used to determine the number of calories used while doing physical activity or any exercise. A *calorie*, or more accurately *kilocalorie* (kcal), is the amount of heat required to raise one liter (1 kg) of water one degree centigrade. In exercise and nutrition the kilocalorie is used exclusively, although often the *kilo* is omitted from the word so that just *calorie* is used to stand for kilocalorie. The fields of chemistry and physics use a small calorie, but this terminology is not used in exercise or nutrition.

The field of study dealing with the caloric cost of exercise is called *calorimetry*. Calorimetry is divided into *direct calorimetry* and *indirect calorimetry*. Direct calorimetry is done in a carefully constructed chamber that is completely insulated from environmental temperature. A subject rests or exercises in the chamber, and the heat the subject produces is measured. Because of the expense of constructing this kind of chamber and the amount and sophistication of the measuring instrumentation, only a couple of direct calorimeters exist in the United States. However, while experiments were being conducted using direct calorimetry, the amount of oxygen used by the subjects was also monitored and a relationship was found between the heat actually produced and the amount of oxygen used. It was observed that for each liter of oxygen a subject used, he or she produced 5 kcal. So instead of having to use an expensive calorimeter, the subject's use of oxygen was measured and multiplied by five to determine the amount of heat produced. This method is called indirect calorimetry. Virtually every exercise physiology laboratory uses indirect calorimetry.

The following simple example will illustrate indirect calorimetry: If a subject running on the treadmill has a steady-state oxygen uptake of 2.5 L · min^{-1} and he or she runs for 12 minutes, how many calories are used? Multiplying 2.5 liters of oxygen per minute by 12 minutes gives us 30 liters of oxygen ($2.5 \times 12 = 30$ L). To convert oxygen to calories, multiply the amount of oxygen used by five. The answer is 150 kcal. You can also arrive at this answer by immediately converting to calories; that is, if 2.5 liters of oxygen per minute is 12.5 calories per minute ($2.5 \times 5 = 12.5$), then 12.5 calories per minute for 12 minutes is 150 kcal ($12.5 \times 12 = 150$).

Two kinds of indirect calorimetry exist: *open-circuit spirometry* and *closed-circuit spirometry*. Closed-circuit spirometry was used by hospitals to measure oxygen uptake because closed circuit required no gas analysis. The patient breathed pure oxygen from a tank with a known quantity of oxygen, and after the expired carbon dioxide was removed chemically, the unused oxygen was returned to the tank (it was a closed circuit). This meant that whatever disappeared from the tank, when expressed per minute, was oxygen uptake. Closed-circuit spirometry is now seldom used. With the advent of high-speed gas analyzers, open-circuit spirometry is now used almost exclusively. It is called open circuit because the subject breathes room air (the system is open to the environment). Because the person is breathing room air, which is a mixture of oxygen, nitrogen, and carbon dioxide, the air must be analyzed for oxygen and carbon dioxide to determine the amount of oxygen breathed in and breathed out.

To illustrate converting oxygen to kilocalories, let's estimate the caloric cost of an exercise class. To do this we must make certain assumptions, but these assumptions can be very realistic and accurate.

The following outline is a fairly typical 45-minute exercise class:

5 minutes of warm-up

15 minutes of muscular strength and endurance

20 minutes of aerobic activity

5 minutes of cool-down

We will make certain assumptions:

- Assume the individual in question has a maximum oxygen uptake of three liters per minute. This assumption is close to the average adult's maximum oxygen uptake.

- Assume the individual knows subjectively what maximum work feels like. Individuals who have done a maximum $\dot{V}O_2$ test know the feeling well. For others, it represents an absolute "all-out" performance and total cardiorespiratory fatigue (not muscular fatigue).

With these assumptions in mind, let's estimate the intensity of each of the program components. We cannot determine exact answers, but with some imagination we can decide upon fairly accurate figures. First we need to decide at what percentage of maximum $\dot{V}O_2$ each of the components of the above exercise class is performed.

- *Warm-up and cool-down.* These two can be combined because they are of similar intensity. At what percentage of maximum is an individual working during a warm-up and cool-down? During a warm-up joints are being put through their full range of movement, mild exercise causes deeper breathing, and the heart rate may increase a little. The warm-up does not cause cardiorespiratory stress. We will use a figure of 10% of maximum oxygen uptake. This figure could be 15% or some other intensity, but 10% is fairly reasonable.

- *Muscular strength and endurance.* Remember we are considering respiratory capacity, not muscular capacity. At what percentage of maximum oxygen uptake is an individual working during the muscular strength and endurance phase? Let's assume these are calisthenics (such as push-ups, crunches, chest raises) and normally participants rest a little between each exercise. Although participants may be working their muscles hard and may be tired, they experience very little cardiorespiratory stress. We will assume 30% of $\dot{V}O_2$max.

- *Aerobic activity.* Because we often ask exercisers to work at 75% of maximum heart rate, we will assume that they are exercising at approximately 75% of their maximum oxygen uptake.

Estimating the caloric cost of this program using these assumptions, we can calculate the following:

- *Warm-up and cool-down.* We estimated these as being 10% of a $\dot{V}O_2$max. Ten percent of three liters (assumed $\dot{V}O_2$max) (0.1 × 3) is 0.3 liter per minute, so during the warm-up and cool-down the amount of oxygen being used is 0.3 liter per minute. If the warm-up and cool-down took 10 minutes, then during 10 minutes 3 liters were totally used (0.3 × 10 = 3 L) To convert to calories, multiply the liters of oxygen used by five, which in this example is 15 kcal. The warm-up and cool-down portions of the class used 15 kcal.

■ *Muscular strength and endurance.* We estimated this part of the workout as being 30% of a $\dot{V}O_2$max. Thirty percent of 3 liters (assumed $\dot{V}O_2$max) (0.3×3) is 0.9 liter per minute, so during the strength and muscular endurance training the amount of oxygen being used is 0.9 liter per minute. If the muscular strength and endurance portion took 15 minutes, then during 15 minutes 13.5 liters were totally used ($0.9 \times 15 = 13.5$ liters). To convert to calories, multiply the liters of oxygen used by five, which in this example is 67.5 kcal. The muscular strength and endurance portion of the class used 67.5 kcal.

■ *Aerobic activity.* We estimated this part of the workout as being 75% of a $\dot{V}O_2$max. Seventy-five percent of 3 liters (assumed $\dot{V}O_2$max) (0.75×3) is 2.25 liters per minute, so during the aerobic portion the amount of oxygen being used is 2.25 liters per minute. If the aerobic portion took 20 minutes, then during those 20 minutes 45 liters were totally used ($2.25 \times 20 = 45$ liters). To convert to calories, multiply the liters of oxygen used by five, which in this example is 225 kcal. The aerobic portion of the class used 225 kcal.

The total caloric cost of this exercise program is estimated at 307.5 kcal ($15 + 67.5 + 225 = 307.5$). The above program was actually measured using open-circuit spirometry and was found to use 291 kcal.

To estimate the caloric cost of an exercise, estimate the percentage of $\dot{V}O_2$max the exercise is using. See table 4.2 for help in estimating exercise intensity.

Table 4.2 Exercise Intensity Classifications

Classification of intensity	RPE	%$\dot{V}O_2$R HR reserve	%Max HR
Very light	<10	<20	<35
Light	10-11	20-39	35-54
Moderate	12-13	40-59	55-69
Hard	14-16	60-84	70-89
Very hard	17-19	85	90
Maximal	20	100	100

Adapted from U.S. Department of Health and Human Services: *Physical Activity and Health: A Report of the Surgeon General.* Atlanta, GA: U.S. Department of Health and Human Service, Centers for Disease Control and Prevention, National Center for Chronic Disease Prevention and Health Promotion, 1996.

Metabolic Equivalent (METS)

A linear relationship exists between heart rate and workload and between $\dot{V}O_2$ and workload. As work increases, the heart rate and oxygen uptake both increase linearly. If these two are both linear with the workload, then a linear relationship must also exist between heart rate and $\dot{V}O_2$ (see figure 4.24).

The top graph in figure 4.24 is the same as the bottom graph except that work has been replaced by $\dot{V}O_2$. If the relationships just described are true, as heart rate goes up, so too does $\dot{V}O_2$, and it does so linearly. $\dot{V}O_2$ can be a measurement of work, and the unit used to express $\dot{V}O_2$ is a *MET*, or *metabolic equivalent*. A MET by definition is the amount of oxygen used at rest. One MET is the amount of oxygen used at rest, so that two METs is twice the oxygen used at rest, five METs is five times the amount of oxygen used at rest, and so on.

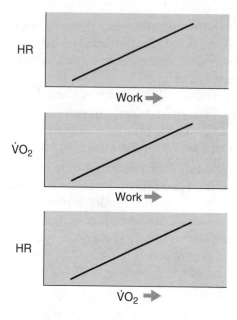

Figure 4.24 Linear relationship between heart rate and $\dot{V}O_2$.

Although work may be expressed as multiples of resting metabolism, we noted earlier that the amount of oxygen a person uses at rest is a function of the individual's size (weight). Larger individuals have larger $\dot{V}O_2$s at rest. The top portion of table 4.3 lists a group of individuals of different weights and their resting $\dot{V}O_2$s.

Individuals carrying more weight have larger resting $\dot{V}O_2$s. Using the definition that work is expressed as multiples of resting metabolism, it would appear from table 4.3 that if John were doing two METs of work, his $\dot{V}O_2$ would be 0.664 L · min⁻¹ ($2 \times 0.332 = 0.664$). By the same token if Jane were doing two METs of work, her $\dot{V}O_2$ would only be 0.316 L · min⁻¹ ($2 \times .158 = .316$).

As mentioned earlier, the amount of work a person is doing ($\dot{V}O_2$) can only be compared to others if their weight is equated. The bottom of table 4.3 equates the participants' weight by dividing the amount of oxygen needed at rest by body weight. What we find is that everyone has the same resting metabolism when expressed per unit of body weight: 3.5 ml/kg/min (ml · kg⁻¹ · min⁻¹). Therefore, when we divide the amount of oxygen a person needs at rest (large or small) by his or her body weight and we express the amount of oxygen used per minute for each pound (or in science, kilogram) of body weight, we find that everyone has the same resting $\dot{V}O_2$. Sharing the same resting $\dot{V}O_2$ equalizes everyone. A large man will express the amount of oxygen he uses at rest, not totally, but for each kilogram of his weight; a small woman expresses the amount of oxygen she uses at rest, not totally, but for each kilogram of her weight. Now we can compare one kilogram of the man's weight to one kilogram of the woman's weight. When we make this comparison, we find that the amount of oxygen used at rest per minute is the same for everyone, 3.5 milliliters of oxygen for every kilogram of body weight per minute (3.5 ml · kg⁻¹ · min⁻¹).

Figure 4.25 shows a 74-kg man at rest. His resting metabolic rate or resting $\dot{V}O_2$ is 0.259 L · min⁻¹ or 259 ml · min⁻¹. This is the amount of oxygen needed through-

Table 4.3 Sample Weights and Resting $\dot{V}O_2$

	Weight	Resting $\dot{V}O_2$
Tom	82kg. (180lbs)	.287L/min.
John	95kg. (209lbs)	.332L/min.
Dick	80kg. (176lbs)	.280L/min.
Harry	70kg. (154lbs)	.245L/min.
Mary	60kg. (132lbs)	.210L/min.
Betty	50kg. (110lbs)	.175L/min.
Jane	45kg. (99lbs)	.158L/min.

Divide by body weight to eliminate the effect of weight.

Tom	287/82	= 3.5ml/kg/min.
John	332/95	= 3.5ml/kg/min.
Dick	280/80	= 3.5ml/kg/min.
Harry	245/70	= 3.5ml/kg/min.
Mary	210/60	= 3.5ml/kg/min.
Betty	175/50	= 3.5ml/kg/min.
Jane	158/45	= 3.5ml/kg/min.

out his body. As he weighs 74 kg, if we divide the total amount of oxygen he uses by his body weight, each kilogram uses 3.5 ml of oxygen per minute.

Now we have a numerical value for a MET: 3.5 ml $\cdot$ kg^{-1} $\cdot$ min^{-1}. The definition has not changed; a MET is still the amount of oxygen used at rest, but because we've made everyone the same weight so we can compare them, the value of resting metabolism is 3.5 ml $\cdot$ kg^{-1} $\cdot$ min^{-1} for everyone. If we express work as METs, it is easy to convert the METs into $\dot{V}O_2$. If one MET is 3.5 ml $\cdot$ kg^{-1} $\cdot$ min^{-1}, then

- 2 METs = 7.0 ml $\cdot$ kg^{-1} $\cdot$ min^{-1} (2 × 3.5 = 7),
- 3 METs = 10.5 ml $\cdot$ kg^{-1} $\cdot$ min^{-1} (3 × 3.5 = 10.5),
- 8 METs = 28 ml $\cdot$ kg^{-1} $\cdot$ min^{-1} (8 × 3.5 = 28), and
- 12 METs = 42 ml $\cdot$ kg^{-1} $\cdot$ min^{-1} (12 × 3.5 = 42).

An example will illustrate: If an 82-kg man is stepping and has a $\dot{V}O_2$ of 2.17 L $\cdot$ min^{-1}, how many METs is he working at? The first thing to do is to express his $\dot{V}O_2$ per kg of body weight because that's how METs are expressed. His $\dot{V}O_2$ was 2.17 L $\cdot$ min^{-1}, which is 2170 ml $\cdot$ min^{-1}. Divide this by his body weight to express his $\dot{V}O_2$ per unit of body weight (2170 ml/82kg), which is 26.46 ml $\cdot$ kg^{-1} $\cdot$ min^{-1}. This means that while he was stepping each kilogram of his body was using 26.46 ml of oxygen. If one MET is 3.5 ml $\cdot$ kg^{-1} $\cdot$ min^{-1}, how many times 3.5 is 26.46? Divide 26.46 by 3.5 to get 7.5 METs. While stepping he was using 7.5 times the amount of oxygen he used at rest.

A note to remember. If you want METs: Take the $\dot{V}O_2$ in liters per minute and express it in ml $\cdot$ kg^{-1} $\cdot$ min^{-1}, then divide by 3.5.

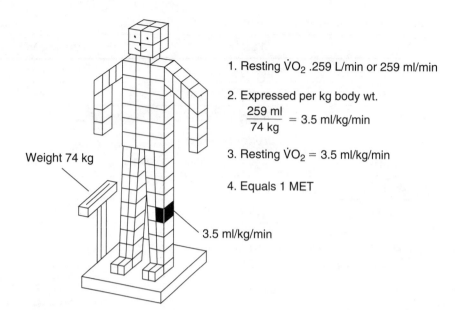

1. Resting $\dot{V}O_2$ .259 L/min or 259 ml/min

2. Expressed per kg body wt.
$$\frac{259 \text{ ml}}{74 \text{ kg}} = 3.5 \text{ ml/kg/min}$$

3. Resting $\dot{V}O_2$ = 3.5 ml/kg/min

4. Equals 1 MET

Weight 74 kg

3.5 ml/kg/min

Figure 4.25   Example of resting metabolic rate.

Here's another example: A 60-kg woman runs on the treadmill at 8 mph and up a 2% grade. Her steady-state $\dot{V}O_2$ is measured at 3.1 L · min⁻¹. How many METs is she working at?

(Follow the directions in the previous note.)

1. Take the $\dot{V}O_2$ and express it in ml · kg⁻¹ · min⁻¹. This equals 51.67 ml · kg⁻¹ · min⁻¹ (3100ml/60kg = 51.67 ml · kg⁻¹ · min⁻¹).

2. How many times greater than rest is this? Divide the $\dot{V}O_2$ in ml · kg⁻¹ by 3.5. She is working at 14.76 METs. (51.67/3.5 = 14.76 METs), which is saying that she is using 14.76 times the amount of oxygen she used at rest.

Practically all recreational and occupational tasks have been measured for metabolic equivalents (METs). Activities that have the same MET value are the same intensity and use the same amount of oxygen (and therefore calories) per minute per kilogram of body weight.

For instance, a man and woman work in the garden and rake leaves. The man is 80 kg and the woman is 50 kg. A MET table tells us that leaf raking has a MET value between three and six METs. For our example let's assume the value is five METs. That means that this task per minute takes five times the amount of oxygen used at rest per minute. We have already determined that everybody uses 3.5 ml of oxygen for each kilogram of body weight per minute at rest. So 5 METs is 5 × 3.5 or 17.5 ml of oxygen per minute for anyone who is raking leaves. The man weighs 80 kg, so he will use totally 1.4 L of oxygen per minute (80 × 17.5 = 1400 = 1.4 L). The woman, who weighs 50 kg, will use 0.875 L of oxygen per minute (50 kg × 17.5 ml = 875 = 0.875 L).

Calories are determined from the amount of oxygen used (indirect calorimetry). If the amount of oxygen used is known, then the oxygen (in liters) is multiplied by five to convert it to calories. Remember that 1000 milliliters equals 1 liter, so milliliter measurements must be divided by 1000 before being multiplied by 5. In the previous example, the man was using 1400 ml of oxygen per minute while raking. If we divide 1400 by 1000, we get 1.4 L; if we multiply 1.4 L by 5, we get the number of calories burned per minute, which is 7 kcal/min (1.4 $\times$ 5 = 7 calories per min). The woman was using 875 ml of oxygen per minute or 0.875 L per minute (875/1000 = 0.875). Multiply by five to calculate the calories. The woman is using 4.4 calories per minute while raking.

The MET level while raking leaves was the same for both the man and the woman, when their $\dot{V}O_2$ was expressed as ml $\cdot$ kg^{-1} $\cdot$ min^{-1}. But when we consider the whole man and the whole woman, $\dot{V}O_2$ must be multiplied by their body weight. Then the $\dot{V}O_2$ is different and so is the caloric cost.

Summary of Metabolic Equivalents (METs)

A MET is the amount of oxygen that is used per minute at rest. But everyone uses a different amount of oxygen per minute at rest because everyone is a different size. A big man has a big heart, big lungs, big body, and big muscles to support posture at rest as well as a bigger digestive system. All of this takes oxygen to operate. A small woman has a smaller body and smaller body systems, and therefore needs less oxygen to operate them.

When the amount of oxygen an individual needs at rest (large or small) is divided by her or his body weight, the amount of oxygen used per minute is expressed for each kilogram of body weight. Divide body weight by 2.2 to get weight in kilograms. For example, a man weighing 180 pounds weighs 81.8 kg (180/2.2), and a woman weighing 110 pounds weighs 50 kg (110/2.2).

Dividing by weight equalizes everyone: A large man expresses the amount of oxygen he uses at rest not totally, but for each kilogram of his weight; a small woman expresses the amount of oxygen she uses at rest not totally, but for each kilogram of her weight. Now we can compare one kilogram of the man's weight to one kilogram of the woman's weight. When we make this comparison, we find that the amount of oxygen used at rest per minute is the same for everyone: 3.5 milliliters of oxygen for every kilogram of body weight per minute (3.5 ml $\cdot$ kg^{-1}). This number is the resting oxygen consumption for everyone (also called *resting metabolism* or *resting oxygen uptake*), and it is one MET.

Work or exercise is expressed as multiples of resting oxygen uptake so that

- 2 METs is twice the amount of oxygen used at rest or 7 ml of oxygen per kg of body weight (2 $\times$ 3.5 = 7),
- 3 METs is three times the amount of oxygen used at rest or 10.5 ml of oxygen per kg of body weight (3 $\times$ 3.5 = 10.5),
- 5 METs is five times the amount of oxygen used at rest or 17.5 ml of oxygen per kg of body weight (5 $\times$ 3.5 = 17.5), and
- 12 METs is twelve times the amount of oxygen used at rest or 42 ml of oxygen per kg of body weight (12 $\times$ 3.5 = 42).

So, if you are exercising at an 8-MET intensity, you are using 28 ml of oxygen per kilogram of body weight per minute (3.5 $\times$ 8 = 28) (and so is *everybody* who is doing 8 METs of work). If you weigh 81.8 kgs (180 lbs), you are using 28 ml of oxygen for every kilogram of weight. Totally you are using 2.29 liters of oxygen per minute (28 ml $\times$ 81.8 kg = 2290.4 ml). The MET intensity can be converted to calories by multiplying the amount of oxygen used by five. In this example, working at 8 METs is using 11.45 calories per minute (2.29 $\times$ 5 = 11.45).

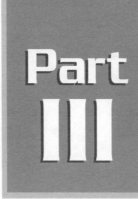

Part III

Fitness Testing at the YMCA

Chapter 5

Introduction to Fitness Testing

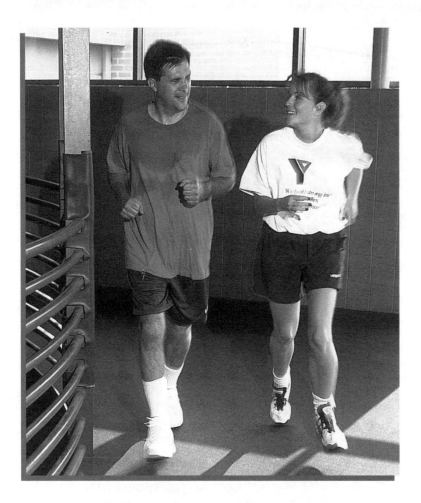

For many exercise program participants, testing and evaluation prior to and at set intervals during participation is important. Testing and evaluation are conducted for the following reasons:

- To assess current fitness levels
- To identify training needs
- To select training regimens
- To evaluate the participant's progress
- To evaluate the success of the program in achieving its objectives
- To motivate participants

The evaluation phase of an exercise program may be divided into two categories: health screening of a participant, which is the responsibility of the individual and his or her physician, and fitness assessment, which is the responsibility of the YMCA fitness director. This chapter describes the difference between health screening and fitness assessments and provides basic information about each. The specific details of the fitness evaluation chosen for the YMCA Fitness Assessment protocol are covered separately in chapter 6. Also included in this chapter is an explanation of reliability in physical fitness testing.

Using YMCA Fitness Analyst

What Is YMCA Fitness Analyst?

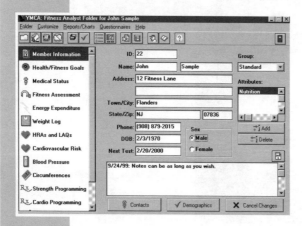

YMCA Fitness Analyst is a software package that can assist you in collecting health and lifestyle information from your members, in recording members' fitness assessment results, and in providing members with feedback on their fitness progress. It automatically performs calculations on the fitness testing data you enter, comparing them to norms and to members' individual test goals. The package generates test result reports, graphs, and charts and provides educational materials, all of which you can print out.

The main screen for the software is the Member Information Page. Here you can record basic information about Y members such as name, address, birth date, gender, phone number, and contact information. You can gain access to all the other features of the software package from this page.

The software enables you to assign each member to a group (such as a particular fitness class) or to an attribute (such as older adults). The ability to categorize allows you to create targeted mailing lists or to print reports summarizing information for particular groupings.

YMCA Fitness Analyst is available through the YMCA Program Store. To see how the software can assist you throughout the fitness assessment and follow-up process, read the "Using YMCA Fitness Analyst" sidebars that highlight how each page of the software can be applied.

Health Screening Versus Physical Fitness Evaluation

The health and fitness director, the Medical Advisory Committee, and the participant need to understand the difference between health screening and physical fitness evaluation. For years fitness directors tested physical fitness before and after training programs to show changes in physical fitness and efficiency. Push-ups, chin-ups, mile runs, agility tests, and step tests were commonly used.

However, when the cycle ergometer and stethoscope were used to evaluate cardiorespiratory fitness, people sometimes viewed the ergometer test as a test of exercise program readiness and not as a test of cardiovascular fitness. Terms such as *stress test* and *diagnosis* were used incorrectly. The result of using these traditionally medical terms was that some individuals misinterpreted the purpose of the test. The cycle ergometer test evaluates cardiorespiratory efficiency by measuring the heart rate while slowly increasing the workloads. The test is given only for evaluation of cardiorespiratory fitness and not for exercise clearance or diagnosis of abnormalities.

The health screening, however, is appropriate for determining readiness of an individual to engage in a fitness testing and/or exercise program. A trained physician may evaluate the electrocardiogram (ECG) and blood pressure of an individual who is exercising on a treadmill. Along with a medical history, an individual's limitations to exercise, if any, are determined. The tests are used to give medical clearance or to diagnose early signs of heart disease but not to determine the level of cardiovascular fitness. This confusion between physical fitness evaluation and health screening needs to be clarified and explained to the medical community, the YMCA Medical Advisory Committee, and most of all to the participants.

Health Screening

The recommendations made for the health screening of an individual are basically the same regardless of the nature of the fitness evaluation format. The health screening precedes the fitness testing program. The participant's physician is responsible for administering the medical evaluation and, if necessary, giving his or her consent for the participant's further evaluation by the YMCA Fitness Assessment protocol. This part of the chapter should be shared with the examining physician.

The American College of Sports Medicine (ACSM) has established guidelines for the health screening of adults prior to participating in fitness testing or exercise programs. Emphasis is placed on the age and health status of the proposed participant. The purposes of the preparticipation health screening include the following:

1. Identification and exclusion of individuals with medical contraindications to exercise

2. Identification of individuals at increased risk for disease because of age, symptoms, and/or risk factors who should undergo a medical evaluation and exercise testing before starting an exercise program

3. Identification of persons with clinically significant disease who should participate in a medically supervised exercise program

4. Identification of individuals with other special needs*

The ACSM divides screened individuals into three categories and suggests that health screening include three major components. We recommend that screening be done prior to any testing.

*Reprinted by permission from American College of Sports Medicine, 2000, *ACSM's guidelines for exercise testing and prescription*, 6th ed. (Baltimore: Lippincott Williams & Wilkins), 22.

Categories of Individuals Tested

According to the ACSM, participants can be classified initially into three risk strata:

1. *Low risk*—Younger individuals* who are asymptomatic and meet no more than one risk factor threshold from table 5.1.

2. *Moderate risk*—Older individuals (men ≥ 45 years of age; women ≥ 55 years of age) or those who meet the threshold for two or more risk factors from table 5.1.

3. *High risk*—Individuals with one or more signs/symptoms listed in table 5.2 or known cardiovascular,[†] pulmonary,[‡] or metabolic[§] disease.

*Men < 45 years of age; women < 55 years of age.
[†]Cardiac, peripheral vascular, or cerebrovascular disease.
[‡]Chronic obstructive pulmonary disease, asthma, interstitial lung disease, or cystic fibrosis.
[§]Diabetes mellitus (types 1 and 2), thyroid disorders, renal or liver disease.

Reprinted by permission from American College of Sports Medicine, 2000, *ACSM's guidelines for exercise testing and prescription*, 6th ed. (Baltimore: Lippincott Williams & Wilkins), 26.

Refer to table 5.3 for the ACSM guidelines for screening of each of these three classifications.

Components of Health Screening

The type and extensiveness of a medical evaluation depends on the physician and the category of the individual participant. The ACSM suggests three major components (medical history, physical examination, and laboratory tests) for the health screening.

Medical History

The medical history is the most important part of the screening. Individuals should be questioned about their medical history as shown in table 5.4.

Table 5.1 Coronary Artery Disease Risk Factor Thresholds for Use With ACSM Risk Stratification*

Risk factors	Defining criteria
Positive	
Family history	Myocardial infarction, coronary revascularization, or sudden death before 55 years of age in father or other male first-degree relative (i.e., brother or son), or before 65 years of age in mother or other female first-degree relative (i.e., sister or daughter)
Cigarette smoking	Current cigarette smoker or those who quit within the previous 6 months
Hypertension	Systolic blood pressure of 140 mmHg or diastolic 90 mmHg, confirmed by measurements on at least two separate occasions, or on antihypertensive medication
Hypercholesterolemia	Total serum cholesterol of >200 mg/dL (5.2 mmol/L) or high-density lipoprotein cholesterol of <35 mg/dL (0.9 mmol/L), or on lipid-lowering medication. If low-density lipoprotein cholesterol is available, use >130 mg/dL (3.4 mmol/L) rather than total cholesterol of >200 mg/dL
Impaired fasting glucose	Fasting blood glucose of 110 mg/dL (6.1 mmol/L) confirmed by measurements on at least two separate occasions (7)
Obesity[†]	Body Mass Index of 30 kg/m^2 (8), or waist girth of >100 cm (9)
Sedentary lifestyle	Persons not participating in a regular exercise program or meeting the minimal physical activity recommendations[‡] from the U.S. Surgeon General's report (10)
Negative	
High serum HDL cholesterol[§]	>60 mg/dL (1.6 mmol/L)

*Adapted from Expert Panel on Detection, Evaluation, and Treatment of High Blood Cholesterol in Adults. Summary of the second report of the National Cholesterol Education Program (NCEP) expert panel on detection, evaluation, and treatment of high blood cholesterol in adults (Adult Treatment Panel II). *JAMA* 1993; 269:3015-3023.

[†]Professional opinions vary regarding the most appropriate markers and thresholds for obesity; therefore, exercise professionals should use clinical judgment when evaluating this risk factor.

[‡]Accumulating 30 minutes or more of moderate physical activity on most days of the week.

[§]It is common to sum risk factors in making clinical judgments. If high-density lipoprotein (HDL) cholesterol is high, subtract one risk factor from the sum of the positive risk factors because high HDL decreases CAD risk.

Table 5.2 Major Symptoms or Signs Suggestive of Cardiovascular and Pulmonary Disease*

1.	Pain, discomfort (or other anginal equivalent) in the chest, neck, jaw, arms, or other areas that may be due to ischemia
2.	Shortness of breath at rest or with mild exertion
3.	Dizziness or syncope
4.	Orthopnea or paroxysmal nocturnal dyspnea
5.	Ankle edema
6.	Palpitations or tachycardia
7.	Intermittent claudication
8.	Known heart murmur
9.	Unusual fatigue or shortness of breath with usual activities

*These symptoms must be interpreted in the clinical context in which they appear because they are not all specific for cardiovascular, pulmonary, or metabolic disease.

Reprinted by permission from American College of Sports Medicine, 2000, *ACSM's guidelines for exercise testing and prescription*, 6th ed. (Baltimore: Lippincott Williams & Wilkins).

Table 5.3 ACSM Recommendations for (A) Current Medical Examination* and Exercise Testing Prior to Participation and (B) Physician Supervision of Exercise Tests

	Low risk	Moderate risk	High risk
A.			
Moderate exercise[†]	Not necessary[‡]	Not necessary	Recommended
Vigorous exercise[§]	Not necessary	Recommended	Recommended
B.			
Submaximal test	Not necessary	Not necessary	Recommended
Maximal test	Not necessary	Recommended[¶]	Recommended

*Within the past year.
[†]Absolute moderate exercise is defined as activities that are approximately 3-6 METs or the equivalent of brisk walking at 3 to 4 mph for most healthy adults (13). Nevertheless, a pace of 3 to 4 mph might be considered "hard" to "very hard" by some sedentary, older persons. Moderate exercise may alternatively be defined as an intensity well within the individual's capacity, one which can be comfortably sustained for a prolonged period of time (~45 min), which has a gradual initiation and progression, and is generally noncompetitive. If an individual's exercise capacity is known, relative moderate exercise may be defined by the range 40-60% maximal oxygen uptake.
[‡]The designation of "Not necessary" reflects the notion that a medical examination, exercise test, and physician supervision of exercise testing would not be essential in the preparticipation screening; however, they should not be viewed as inappropriate.
Vigorous exercise is defined as activities of >6 METs. Vigorous exercise may alternatively be defined as exercise intense enough to represent a substantial cardiorespiratory challenge. If an individual's exercise capacity is known, vigorous exercise may be defined as an intensity of >60% maximal oxygen uptake.
[¶]When physician supervision of exercise testing is "Recommended," the physician should be in close proximity and readily available should there be an emergent need.
Reprinted by permission from American College of Sports Medicine, 2000, *ACSM's guidelines for exercise testing and prescription*, 6th ed. (Baltimore: Lippincott Williams & Wilkins,) 27.

Table 5.4 Components of the Medical History

---

1. **Medical diagnosis**—cardiovascular disease including myocardial infarction; percutaneous coronary artery procedures including angioplasty, coronary stent(s), and atherectomy; coronary artery bypass surgery; valvular surgery(s) and valvular dysfunction (e.g., aortic stenosis/mitral valve disease); other cardiac surgeries such as left ventricular aneurysmectomy and cardiac transplantation; pacemaker and/or implantable cardioverter defibrillator; presence of aortic aneurysm; ablation procedures for arrhythmias; symptoms of ischemic coronary syndrome (angina pectoris); peripheral vascular disease; hypertension; diabetes; obesity; pulmonary disease including asthma, emphysema, and bronchitis; cerebrovascular disease including stroke and transient ischemic attacks; anemia and other blood dyscrasias (e.g., lupus erythematosis); phlebitis, deep vein thrombosis or emboli; cancer; pregnancy; osteoporosis; musculoskeletal disorders; emotional disorders; eating disorders

---

2. **Previous physical examination findings**—murmurs, clicks, gallop rhythms, other abnormal heart sounds, and other unusual cardiac and vascular findings; abnormal pulmonary findings (e.g., wheezes, rales, crackles); abnormal blood sugar, blood lipids, and lipoproteins, or other significant laboratory abnormalities; high blood pressure; edema

---

3. **History of symptoms**—discomfort (pressure, tingling, pain, heaviness, burning, tightness, squeezing, numbness) in the chest, jaw, neck, back, or arms; lightheadedness, dizziness, or fainting; temporary loss of visual acuity or speech, transient unilateral numbness or weakness; shortness of breath; rapid heart beats or palpitations, especially if associated with physical activity, eating a large meal, emotional upset, or exposure to cold (or any combination of these activities)

---

4. **Recent illness, hospitalization, new medical diagnoses, or surgical procedures**

---

5. **Orthopedic problems**, including arthritis; joint swelling; any condition that would make ambulation or use of certain test modalities difficult

---

6. **Medication use, drug allergies**

---

7. **Other habits**, including caffeine, alcohol, tobacco, or recreational (illicit) drug use

---

8. **Exercise history**—information on readiness for change and habitual level of activity: type of exercise, frequency, duration, and intensity

---

9. **Work history** with emphasis on current or expected physical demands, noting upper and lower extremity requirements

---

10. **Family history** of cardiac, pulmonary, or metabolic disease, stroke, sudden death

---

Reprinted by permission from American College of Sports Medicine, 2000, *ACSM's guidelines for exercise testing and prescription*, 6th ed. (Baltimore: Lippincott Williams & Wilkins), 36.

Using YMCA Fitness Analyst

Collecting Medical Status Information

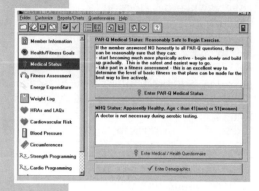

Medical Health Questionnaire

This form asks you a variety of questions about your medical condition and takes about 5 minutes to complete. We do ask some demographic questions in order to help us with ongoing research. Your answers to these questions will be maintained in privacy and will not be associated with your name in any research. Please fill in the information requested, or place a check in the appropriate space. We thank you for your time and effort in completing this questionnaire.

Please print your name: _____

Today's date: ____/____/____

Please circle the highest grade in school you have completed:
Elementary School 1 2 3 4 5 6 7 8
High School 9 10 11 12
College/Postgrad 13 14 15 16 17 18 19 20+

What is your marital status? ___ Single   ___ Married
                             ___ Widowed   ___ Divorced/Separated

What is your race or ethnic background?
___ White, not of Hispanic origin   ___ American Indian/Alaskan native
___ Asian   ___ Black, not of Hispanic origin
___ Pacific Islander   ___ Hispanic

What is your job or occupation?
(Check the one that applies to the greatest percentage of your time.)
___ Health professional   ___ Disabled, unable to work   ___ Service
___ Manager, educator, professn'l ___ Operator, fabricator, laborer
Unemployed
___ Skilled crafts   ___ Homemaker   ___ Student
___ Technical, sales, support   ___ Retired   ___ Other

How long have you exercised or played sports regularly?
___ I do not exercise regularly   ___ less than 1 year   ___ 1 to 2 years
___ 2 to 5 years   ___ 5 to 10 years   ___ more than 10 years

Known Diseases
❑ 1. Do you have any personal history of heart disease?
❑ 2. Any personal history of metabolic disease (thyroid,renal,liver)?
❑ 3. Have you had diabetes for less than 15 years?
❑ 4. Have you had diabetes for 15 years or more?

The Medical Status page helps you gather information about a member's health history and current lifestyle habits so you can assess the member's readiness for both fitness testing and exercise prescription. It includes the PAR-Q screening form, which will help you determine if the member has any health problems that would prohibit exercise testing or exercise, and a Medical/Health Questionnaire (MHQ) for gathering more detailed health information.

The PAR-Q shows the results on the screen immediately.

The MHQ includes questions on the following:

- Symptoms or signs suggestive of disease
- Chronic disease risk factors
- Medical screening history (both general questions and questions specifically for men or women)
- Listing of medications taken regularly
- Work environment

Once the MHQ is completed, you can print out a summary that will highlight problem areas.

For more in-depth health information about a member, you can have the member fill out additional health risk assessments (HRAs) or lifestyle assessment questionnaires (LAQs).

If you have the Standard Edition of YMCA Fitness Analyst, you will have the following forms available:

- YMCA Health Check*
- YMCA Lifestyle Assessment Questionnaire
- Framingham Cardiovascular Heart Disease Risk Analysis

If you have the Comprehensive Edition, you also will have these additional forms:

- American Cancer Society Dietary Risk Profile
- Arizona Women's Heart Risk Assessment
- ASU (Appalachian State University) Heart Check
- Diabetes Risk Assessment Scale from the American Diabetes Association
- General Lifestyle Questionnaire

YMCA Health Check Questionnaire

This form asks you a variety of questions about your lifestyle habits, and takes about 5 minutes to complete. Please fill in the information requested, or place a check in the appropriate space. We thank you for your time and effort in completing this questionnaire.

Personal Information

Today's date: _____/_____/_____

Please print your name: _____

Age: _____ yrs;   Sex (Circle one):   Male   Female

Demographics

Please circle the highest grade in school you have completed:
Elementary School   1   2   3   4   5   6   7   8
High School   9   10   11   12
College/Postgrad   13   14   15   16   17   18   19   20+

What is your marital status?   ___ Single   ___ Married
                                ___ Widowed   ___ Divorced/Separated

What is your race or ethnic background?
___ White, not of Hispanic origin   ___ American Indian/Alaskan native
___ Asian   ___ Black, not of Hispanic origin
___ Pacific Islander   ___ Hispanic

What is your job or occupation?
(Check the one that applies to the greatest percentage of your time.)
___ Health professional   ___ Disabled, unable to work
___ Service   ___ Manager, educator, professn'l
___ Operator, fabricator, laborer ___ Unemployed
___ Skilled crafts   ___ Homemaker
___ Student   ___ Technical, sales, support
___ Retired   ___ Other

Height and Weight

How tall are you? _____ feet & inches

How much do you weigh (minimal clothing and without shoes)? _____ lbs

What is the most you have ever weighed? _____ lbs

Lifestyle Assessment Questionnaire

This form asks you a variety of questions about your lifestyle habits, and takes about 10 minutes to complete. Please fill in the information requested, or place a check in the appropriate space. We thank you for your time and effort in completing this questionnaire.

Personal Information

Today's date: _____/_____/_____

Please print your name: _____

Age: _____ yrs;   Height: _____ feet & inches

Weight: _____ lbs   Sex (Circle one): Male   Female

Please circle the highest grade in school you have completed:
Elementary School   1   2   3   4   5   6   7   8
High School   9   10   11   12
College/Postgrad   13   14   15   16   17   18   19   20+

What is your marital status?   ___ Single   ___ Married
                                ___ Widowed   ___ Divorced/Separated

What is your race or ethnic background?
___ White, not of Hispanic origin   ___ American Indian/Alaskan native
___ Asian   ___ Black, not of Hispanic origin
___ Pacific Islander   ___ Hispanic

What is your job or occupation?
(Check the one that applies to the greatest percentage of your time.)
___ Health professional   ___ Disabled, unable to work   ___ Service
___ Manager, educator, professn'l ___ Operator, fabricator, laborer ___
Unemployed
___ Skilled crafts   ___ Homemaker   ___ Student
___ Technical, sales, support ___ Retired   ___ Other

Health
Health is defined as a state of complete physical, mental, social, and spiritual well-being, and not merely the absence of disease and infirmity.

1. Please rate how important your health is to you:
   1_ 2_ 3_ 4_ 5_ 6_ 7_ 8_ 9_ 10_
   Not at all   Somewhat   Extremely
   important   important   important

2. In general, compared to other persons your age, rate how healthy you are:
   1_ 2_ 3_ 4_ 5_ 6_ 7_ 8_ 9_ 10_
   Not at all   Somewhat   Extremely
   healthy   healthy   healthy

- General Well-Being Scale
- Michigan Alcoholism Screening Test
- Osteoporosis Risk Checklist

You can print the YMCA Health Check or the YMCA Lifestyle Assessment results individually. All HRA results are printed out as part of a Comprehensive Report of Findings.

*Adapted, by permission, from Loma Linda University Medical Center, Center for Health Promotion, Employee Wellness Questionnaire. Prepared by Dr. David Abbey, Research Director.

Physical Examination

A limited physical examination is useful for specially assessing individuals. It should include the components shown in table 5.5.

Laboratory Tests

Laboratory data are important in making the determination of whether an individual fits into the higher risk category. Some laboratory data are helpful prior to testing those with known cardiac, pulmonary, or metabolic disease. The tests mentioned in table 5.6 are useful in assessing risk and in assigning individuals to the categories described.

Table 5.5 Components of the Physical Examination

Body weight; in many instances, determination of body mass index (BMI), waist-to-hip ratio, waist girth, and/or body composition (percent body fat) is desirable
Apical pulse rate and rhythm
Resting blood pressure, seated, supine, and standing
Auscultation of the lungs with specific attention to uniformity of breath sounds in all areas (absence of rales, wheezes, and other breathing sounds)
Palpation of the cardiac apical impulse—PMI (point of maximal impulse)
Auscultation of the heart with specific attention to murmurs, gallops, clicks, and rubs
Palpation and auscultation of carotid, abdominal, and femoral arteries
Evaluation of the abdomen for bowel sounds, masses, visceromegaly, tenderness
Palpation and inspection of lower extremities for edema and presence of arterial pulses
Absence or presence of tendon xanthoma and skin xanthelasma
Follow-up examination related to orthopedic or other medical conditions that would limit exercise testing
Tests of neurologic function, including reflexes and cognition (as indicated)
Inspection of the skin, especially of the lower extremities in known diabetics

Reprinted by permission from American College of Sports Medicine, 2000, *ACSM's guidelines for exercise testing and prescription,* 6th ed. (Baltimore: Lippincott Williams & Wilkins), 37.

Table 5.6 Recommended Laboratory Tests by Level of Risk and Clinical Assessment

Apparently healthy or individuals at increased risk but without known disease
Total serum cholesterol and HDL cholesterol; other lipoproteins as indicated
Fasting blood glucose, especially in individuals 45 years and younger individuals who are obese (BMI of 30 kg/m ^{2}), have a first-degree relative with diabetes, are members of a high-risk ethnic population (e.g., African-American, Hispanic, Native American), have delivered a baby weighing >9 lbs, or have been diagnosed with gestational diabetes, are hypertensive, have an HDL cholesterol of 35 mg/dL, or on a previous test have had impaired glucose tolerance
Fasting triglycerides, if individual has an elevated total cholesterol, two or more CAD risk factors, diabetes, central obesity, hypertension, chronic renal failure, or suspected familial dyslipidemia. Also consider measuring triglycerides in women on hormone replacement therapy and in persons reporting or known to have a high alcohol intake
Thyroid function, as a screening evaluation especially if dyslipidemia is present
Patients with cardiovascular disease
Above tests plus pertinent previous cardiovascular laboratory tests (e.g., resting 12-lead ECG, Holter monitoring, coronary angiography, radionuclide or echocardiography studies, previous exercise tests)
Carotid ultrasound and other peripheral vascular studies
Consider measures of homocysteine, Lp(a), fibrinogen, LDL particle size (especially in young persons with a strong family history of CAD and in those persons without traditional coronary risk factors)

Patients with pulmonary disease

Chest radiograph, if congestive heart failure is present or suspected

Comprehensive blood chemistry panel and complete blood count as indicated by history and physical examination

Chest radiograph

Pulmonary function tests

Other specialized pulmonary studies (e.g., oximetry or blood gas analysis)

Reprinted by permission from American College of Sports Medicine, 2000, *ACSM's guidelines for exercise testing and prescription*, 6th ed. (Baltimore: Lippincott Williams & Wilkins), 38.

Testing and Exercise Restrictions

The YMCA of the USA recommends that health screening and informed consent forms be required of participants before physical fitness testing begins. The informed consent form should include a statement, signed by the participant, that clearly describes both the testing and the exercise program so that the participant is fully aware of what tests will be given and in what type of exercise he or she will participate. Additionally, a statement of the physician's approval for fitness testing should be included if needed. Sample forms are in appendix A.

The physician, the YMCA Medical Advisory Committee, and the fitness director should also be aware of the relative contraindications to exercise. Individuals having one or more of the contraindications (according to ACSM guidelines) should not be permitted to enter any exercise program without medical approval. Each participant with contraindications should have an individual follow-up in which the benefits of the exercise program are weighed against any resulting harm. Obviously, this demands good clinical judgment. In some instances the participant's condition may not be tangibly altered, but some signs of mental or physical improvement that enhance a sense of well-being may show through. Under such circumstances, the exercise program should be continued even though, from an objective standpoint, the participant's condition remains unchanged.

Physical Fitness Evaluation

After the health screening has been completed and the necessary forms have been received, the participant is ready for the fitness assessment. A typical fitness assessment consists of both standard physical measurements and selected tests that will measure the main components of physical fitness. A certified YMCA Fitness Specialist should perform this evaluation. For participants in their first year of training, it is desirable to repeat the test battery after about 10 to 12 weeks and then again after 6 to 12 months. Repeating the test battery allows participants to observe their personal response to training. After the first year, most participants need not be tested more than once a year.

Participants should be told the following guidelines before they come for fitness testing:

1. Wear exercise clothing and shoes for the test.
2. Do not eat for two hours before testing (this includes drinking coffee or tea).
3. Do not consume alcohol for 24 hours before testing.
4. Do not smoke for two hours before testing.
5. Do not exercise on the day of testing.

Standard Measurements

Measurements of height, weight, and resting heart rate and blood pressure provide a baseline for measuring improvement and evaluating changes. Follow these procedures to record them.

■ *Standing height*. The participant should stand barefoot with the heels together, then stretch upward to the fullest extent. Heels, buttocks, and the upper back should touch a vertical upright such as a wall. The chin should not be lifted. Measurement is recorded in inches (or centimeters) to the nearest quarter-inch. (Because this is not a physical fitness measurement, it may be eliminated. However, it is a good description of the participant and is easy to administer.)

■ *Weight*. Weight should be recorded with the individual wearing shorts, T-shirt, and no shoes. Make note of any deviation from this dress. Record weight in both pounds and kilograms. If recording weight in pounds, record to the nearest quarter-pound.

■ *Resting heart rate*. The resting heart rate should be counted through the use of a stethoscope for one minute. The individual should be sitting (as for a blood-pressure test) and should have had an adequate rest period prior to this test. Adequate rest is indicated when the heart rate has stabilized at a low rate and has not changed.

■ *Resting blood pressure*. The individual sits upright in a straight-backed chair. Both feet are flat on the floor, and the left arm is resting on a table with the elbow flexed. The position is relaxed and comfortable, and the individual is allowed to relax for a few minutes in this position. Conversation is discouraged. The blood pressure is measured with a device called a sphygmomanometer and with a stethoscope. A wide, adjustable cuff is placed around the upper portion of the subject's left arm approximately at heart level. Air is pumped into this cuff, which then expands and presses against the arm to close off the brachial artery, which runs along the inside of the arm. The pressure in the cuff is shown by the sphygmomanometer in millimeters of mercury and initially is pumped up to 200 mmHg, which is normally higher than the individual's blood pressure. The stethoscope is placed in the antecubital space below the cuff. Once the brachial artery has been closed off, air is slowly released from the cuff, and the tester listens for the moment at which the resumption of blood flow can be heard. This resumed flow is characterized by a distinctive sound and is called the *systolic pressure*. The pressure in the cuff is further reduced until blood runs freely through the artery. This point is characterized by the complete disappearance of sound and is called *diastolic pressure*. Three intermediary phases of subtle changes are of little concern here. The first phase, systolic pressure, and the fifth phase, diastolic pressure, should be recorded in millimeters of mercury (mmHg) as indicated on the sphygmomanometer scale.

Physical Fitness Measurements

The four areas of physical fitness typically evaluated in any assessment protocol are body composition, cardiorespiratory endurance, flexibility, and muscular strength and endurance. Numerous tests are available that evaluate these various physical fitness components. For consistency and reliability, the YMCA has chosen field tests that can be administered by virtually any trained YMCA fitness director, and the Y has been using the same test protocol for 30 years. Chapter 6 explains in detail the YMCA's protocol for testing these areas.

Using YMCA Fitness Analyst

Recording Assessment Results

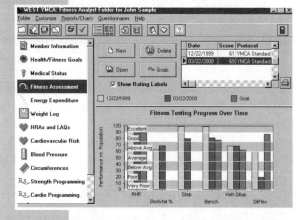

The Fitness Assessment page allows you to collect all the results of your fitness assessments in one convenient place. It records when tests were done and summarizes them on a bar graph that can be printed out.

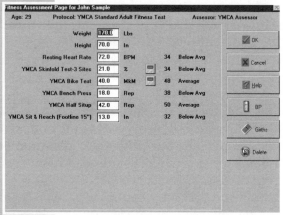

Besides the results of the fitness tests, you also can record the member's height, weight, resting heart rate, and resting blood pressure.

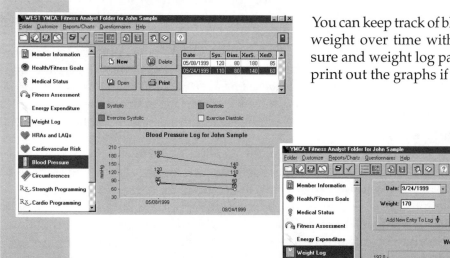

You can keep track of blood pressure and weight over time with the blood pressure and weight log pages, and you can print out the graphs if desired.

Reliability in Physical Fitness Testing

Physical fitness tests are used to evaluate fitness levels. Participants in exercise programs are usually evaluated at the beginning of the program and then again at some future time to assess any physiological changes that have occurred. For test results to be valid, the test battery itself must be reliable. If, for example, on three consecutive days, a pectoral skinfold measured 20 mm, 28 mm, and 36 mm respectively, the differences in the measurements do not reflect changes in the amount of fat, but instead error in the measurement itself. For a test to reflect actual physiological changes, the measurement must be reliable; that is, if a skinfold is measured 10 times over a short period of time, the measurements should be the same or very similar.

The statistical technique that determines the reliability (r) of a measurement is the test-retest reliability coefficient. This reliability coefficient is the correlation between measurements taken on an identical population on two subsequent days. It is an indicator of the reproducibility of a measurement.

Reliability tests can be determined for either a test item or the person administering the test. For a test that is simple to administer (e.g., the flexibility test), a test-retest reliability coefficient can be determined for the test itself. Regardless of who is administering the test, if he or she follows the instructions, procedures, and precautions and has had some supervised practice, the test results should be reliable.

When the test administrator needs additional skills and techniques for a more complicated test, a test-retest reliability coefficient must be determined for each test administrator. The test item may be reliable, but only when measured by a skilled tester. In the YMCA test protocol the skinfold measurements are the only tests that need a reliability coefficient calculated for each tester. Other tests, such as exercise heart rate, resting heart rate, and blood pressure, must be practiced and standardized procedures must be followed, but once these are mastered, they produce reliable measurements. A reliability coefficient can be determined for any test or any tester.

Since we use the term *correlation* frequently, a short review on correlations may be valuable. A simple correlation between two measurements will give the similarity of the two measurements. *To do test reliability, an interclass correlation should be performed. This requires more statistical knowledge; for those interested in learning how to do this, a beginning statistics text can teach the steps involved in an interclass reliability coefficient.*

Correlations can be either positive or negative and they range from perfect positive correlation (+1.00) to perfect negative correlation (–1.00). Table 5.7 shows the range of correlations with general descriptions for each correlation.

Correlations can be either positive or negative, but because negative correlations are not pertinent to test reliability, we discuss only positive correlations. Perfect positive correlation is expressed as +1.0 and is displayed on a graph as a straight line (figure 5.1). For example, if a measurement (e.g., abdominal skinfold) is taken on 25 people and repeated the following day, each measurement would be the same.

Table 5.7 Reliability Coefficients

Correlation (r)	Description
+1.00	Perfect positive correlation
+0.90	Excellent r
+0.80	Good r
+0.70	
+0.60	Fair r
+0.50	
+0.40	Poor r
+0.30	
+0.20	
+0.10	
00.00	No correlation
−0.10	
−0.20	Poor r
−0.30	
−0.40	
−0.50	Fair r
−0.60	
−0.70	Good r
−0.80	
−0.90	Excellent r
−1.00	Perfect negative correlation

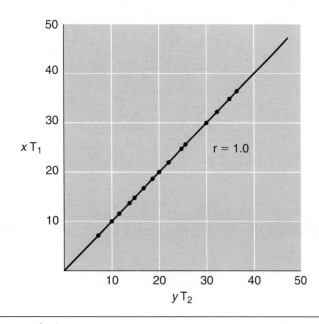

Figure 5.1 Perfect positive correlation.

Perfect correlations in physical fitness testing never occur, but they should be close. Using the example in the previous paragraph, if the abdominal skinfolds taken two days apart were as follows, the correlation would be very good.

T_1	T_2	Difference
18 mm	19 mm	1 mm
25 mm	24 mm	1 mm
30 mm	29 mm	1 mm
10 mm	12 mm	2 mm
12 mm	14 mm	2 mm
15 mm	13 mm	2 mm
22 mm	20 mm	2 mm
24 mm	22 mm	2 mm
31 mm	28 mm	3 mm
30 mm	30 mm	0 mm

These scores are close, perhaps 1 or 2 mm either way. The correlation for this data would be high, which is very good, and if those scores were plotted on graph paper it would look like figure 5.2.

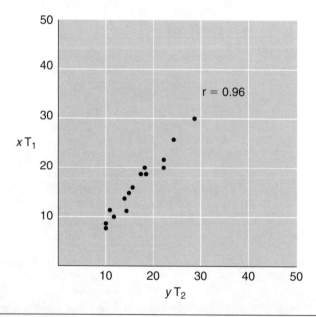

Figure 5.2 The graph is still very linear, showing a very good relationship or reproducibility, but not a straight line.

The farther apart the measurements are, the more the plot points on the graph are scattered and vary. If the abdominal skinfolds taken two days apart were as follows, the correlation would be only fair to poor.

T₁	T₂	Difference
20 mm	15 mm	5 mm
15 mm	20 mm	5 mm
30 mm	25 mm	5 mm
32 mm	25 mm	7 mm
18 mm	20 mm	2 mm
12 mm	24 mm	12 mm
21 mm	28 mm	7 mm
19 mm	24 mm	5 mm
36 mm	28 mm	8 mm
24 mm	19 mm	5 mm

These measurements are farther apart—as much as 12 mm. This correlation is poor and is shown in figure 5.3.

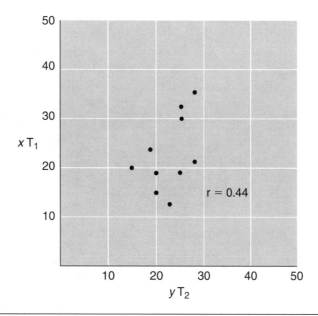

Figure 5.3 The correlation here is poor.

Figure 5.3 shows *some* relationship but it is not very good. An abdominal skinfold of 12 mm one day and 24 mm the next day is poor. If the two measurements of abdominal skinfolds differ widely, there is no relationship. If the data were as follows, the correlation would be poor.

T_1	T_2	Difference
20 mm	14 mm	6 mm
15 mm	21 mm	6 mm
30 mm	24 mm	6 mm
32 mm	25 mm	7 mm
18 mm	25 mm	7 mm
12 mm	24 mm	12 mm
21 mm	28 mm	7 mm
19 mm	26 mm	7 mm
36 mm	25 mm	11 mm
24 mm	15 mm	9 mm

The correlation for this data is very poor, showing no reproducibility. See figure 5.4.

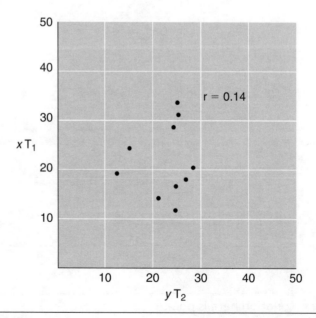

Figure 5.4 The correlation for this data is very poor.

The examples shown here have, for convenience, used just 10 subjects. The minimum number of subjects should be 15; 25 or 30 subjects would be much better. If an abdominal skinfold measurement is taken on 25 people and repeated the following day, each measurement should be almost the same.

Test-retest correlations for skinfolds need to be done on each of the seven sites used in the YMCA test protocol. It is possible to be reliable on one skinfold measurement and not on another. Skinfolds should not be used to evaluate body composition until test-retest reproducibility is good. Using a simple linear correlation, each site should be above 0.90.

The tester does not need to have as much skill for the other tests in the Fitness Assessment protocol, and as long as the tester carefully follows the protocol and first practices under supervision, the test-retest reliabilities of the tests are relatively constant. These are usually done as research studies and are published.

It's important to follow the test's protocol. If, for example, a tester administers the bench-press test, he or she might encourage the participant to really try hard. The participant extends himself and goes to maximum with 15.5 reps. The next week a different tester might give the same subject the bench-press test. This tester offers the participant little encouragement, so the subject stops with 12 reps. This is poor test reliability; if the second tester had encouraged the participant, he might have repeated the 15.5 reps.

Test-retest reliability is equally true of the flexibility test and the crunch test. Participants must be encouraged to go to maximum or the test-retest reliability will not be good. As a practical hint, tests that end on whole numbers are always suspect. Good tests usually end with a half or a quarter of a rep.

Table 5.8 presents the test-retest reliability for each of the tests in the YMCA test protocol. Experienced, conscientious testers did the reliability tests. Due to diurnal fluctuations, the test-retest reliability for blood pressure and resting heart rate were done one hour apart. Both of these measurements tend to change from day to day and even from hour to hour. This is not poor test reliability but fluctuating measurements.

Table 5.8 Reliability of Physical Fitness Tests*

Test item	Correlation
Height	0.99
Weight	0.99
Blood pressure	0.96
Resting HR	0.95
Flexibility	0.94
PWC max	0.95
Timed sit-ups	0.92
3-min step test	0.90

* At the time of this book's publication, these results were at press but were done repeatedly over several years at the University of Nevada at Las Vegas.

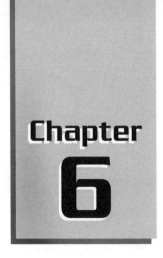

Chapter 6

The YMCA Fitness Assessment Protocol

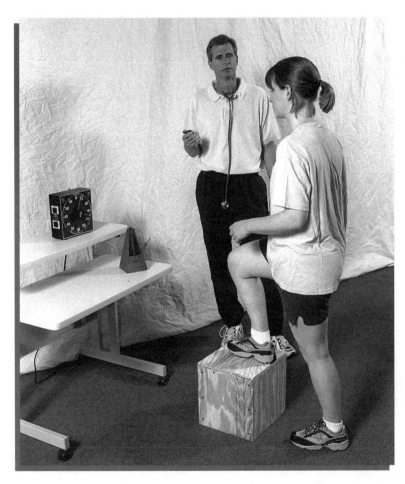

The sophistication and complexity of a fitness testing and assessment program can vary greatly. For many years YMCA fitness programs ranged from no testing at all to testing of practically everything, depending on the individual. Most YMCAs are not prepared to utilize tests that require extensive equipment or advanced training for their administration and interpretation. The YMCA of the USA recommends using those tests that offer valid data about the fitness components being measured.

For these reasons the tests selected for the YMCA Fitness Assessment proto[c] meet the following criteria:

- Minimal amount of testing time for maximal amount of fitness i[n]

- Minimal equipment expenditure required
- Within the capability of the fitness director
- Simple to administer and interpret
- Clearly reflect changes in physical fitness

Beyond the standard YMCA assessments, additional tests and screenings may be used at the discretion of the local YMCA Medical Advisory Committee.

The four areas of physical fitness selected for evaluation in the YMCA Fitness Assessment protocol are body composition, cardiorespiratory endurance, flexibility, and muscular strength and endurance, administered in that order. Here are the specific tests:

1. Body composition—Sum of Four Skinfolds (or Alternate Three)
2. Cardiovascular evaluation—Cycle Ergometer Submaximal Test or Three-Minute Step Test
3. Flexibility measurement—Sit-and-Reach Trunk Flexibility Test
4. Muscular strength and endurance—Bench Press Test and One-Minute Timed Half Sit-Up Test

The tests should be recorded on the score sheet for men or the score sheet for women in appendix B. Be sure to complete the demographic information at the top of the score sheet. Results can then be transferred to the Body Composition Profile and Physical Fitness Evaluation Profile forms that also appear in appendix B. The Physical Fitness Evaluation Profile form rates all results on a scale from excellent to very poor, accompanied by percentile rankings.

Using YMCA Fitness Analyst

Recording and Reporting Assessment Results

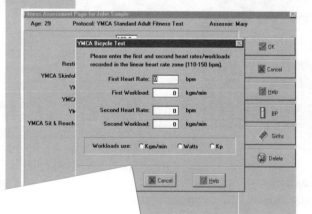

On the Fitness Assessment scoring page, you can enter all the raw data from your member's testing. The page has built-in calculators and pop-up screens that do all the calculations for you. The page also automatically selects and displays the ranking for each score.

continued

Using YMCA Fitness Analyst, *continued*

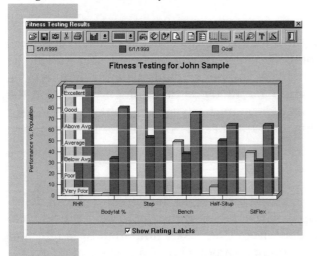

Besides allowing you to record all the results of fitness testing, YMCA Fitness Analyst provides you with the ability to print out reports summarizing those results in a number of ways:

- All Fitness Tests: Change Over Time
- All Fitness Tests: One Date
- Summary Score: Change Over Time
- Single Fitness Test Rank: Change Over Time
- Single Fitness Test Raw Score: Change Over Time

Body Composition and Its Measurement

Body composition refers to lean body weight plus fat weight, which together make up total body weight. The measurement of body composition is important because it can determine the degree of obesity, which is a known health hazard. Obesity is related to a higher incidence of numerous diseases, including coronary heart disease, diabetes, cirrhosis of the liver, hernia, and intestinal obstruction. Many view obesity as a considerable concern from an aesthetic standpoint, and this concern may be one of the primary reasons an obese individual decides to join an exercise program. It is desirable, therefore, to be able to measure an individual's initial body composition before training so as to be able to quantify any change that may occur with training and/or diet. A desirable weight should be determined for the individual, and reducing weight should result from a combination of diet and exercise. Studies have shown that exercise combined with diet guarantees the loss of fat by itself, whereas diet alone results in a loss of fat as well as lean body weight or muscle.

Body weight is not a good measurement of body composition. Height and weight tables are limited because they do not take into consideration what makes up the weight. One person who is 6-feet tall and weighs 200 pounds may be overweight or obese, whereas another person with the same height and weight may be healthy. If the added pounds are fat, this is undesirable; however, if the weight is muscle mass, as in an athlete or a bodybuilder, the extra pounds are healthy and desirable.

In the rest of this section we describe some of the many methods for determining desirable weight or body composition, discuss prediction equations and how percent body fat relates to target weight, and explain how to estimate body fat with skinfold measurements.

Methods of Determining Desirable Weight and Body Composition

Most body composition studies follow the two-compartment model. In this model the body is considered in two compartments: one compartment is fat, and all the rest is considered lean body weight. A number of methods exist to determine what an individual should weigh. Some methods determine a weight on the basis of norm tables and other methods on the basis of a desirable percentage of fat. Each method has its benefits and drawbacks. Some of the most common methods follow.

Height and Weight Tables

Height and weight tables have been used for years as the standard way of determining the desirable body weight. These tables can be read very quickly, are easy to understand, and are widely used. The major limitation of height and weight tables is that they do not distinguish among bone, muscle, and fat. A case demonstrating this limitation occurred in a large metropolitan police department that had height and weight limitations for its officers (which now are considered discriminatory). The maximum allowable weight for a 6-feet tall officer was 210 pounds; above this weight an officer was considered to be overweight and thus subject to suspension. Two officers were suspended for being 6-feet tall and over 210 pounds; both were regular strength training participants and had only 19% fat. Considerable explanation was needed to reinstate the officers. This case clearly illustrates the limitations of height and weight tables.

Tables have been improved by allowing for variations in small, average, and large frames and removing the factors that permitted an increase in weight with age. Because bone and muscle growth is complete when one reaches adulthood, increase in weight with age is mostly due to the accumulation of fat. The same standards are now used for everyone over 25 years of age.

The benefits of the height and weight tables are speed and familiarity. These tables were constructed from data on thousands of people and thus represent good averages. Height and weight is a fast way of crudely describing an individual.

Underwater Weighing*

Underwater, or hydrostatic, weighing is considered to be the gold standard for estimating the amount of fat in the body. Actually, underwater weighing determines body density from which percent body fat can be estimated. The method is based on the physics principle that mass divided by volume equals density. Weight is substituted for mass, and volume is either measured directly (volumetric method) or calculated from Archimedes' Principle, which states that the weight a body loses underwater equals the weight of the water it displaces. From this, one can calculate the volume of the water displaced, which is the volume of the subject. For example, if a 70-kg man weighs 5 kg underwater, his body has displaced 65 kg of water (weight in air minus weight under water or $70 - 5 = 65$ kg). Because one kilogram of water is one liter of water then 65 kilograms is

*Adapted by permission from J. Donahue, L. Golding, and L. Cummings, 1988, "A comparative review of four methods for calculating percent body fat," *Perspective* 14.

equal to 65 liters. The man's density is his weight in the air (70 kg), divided by the weight in air minus the weight in the water (70 − 5 = 65) (70/65 =1.0769). Because some individuals may float or be extremely light in the water, making the obtaining of a weight difficult, a weighted jacket of about 40 pounds is usually fitted on the subject to make him or her heavy. After the weighing the weight of the jacket is subtracted from the underwater weight to give the actual underwater weight.

Two corrections need to be applied when using underwater weighing. First, the density of water changes with temperature, thus affecting the calculation of the volume of the water displaced. Second, any air in the body should be subtracted from the underwater weight. Air comes from two sources in the body: air in the gastrointestinal tract and residual air in the lungs. Gastrointestinal air has been estimated to be approximately 100 ml; this small amount is often dropped from many calculations. The lung residual volume, however, is significant and must be measured to correct the underwater weight.

Usually, underwater weighing is done after the subject has exhaled maximally so that it is only necessary to measure the residual volume. In many laboratories residual volume is measured before the subject steps into the water tank. Once measured, it is assumed that when the subject exhales maximally underwater the same residual volume exists. Exhaling all the air before going underwater is unnatural, uncomfortable, and time limited. In addition, it is questionable as to whether the volume measured on land is the same as the volume in water. A better method is to measure the volume of air in the lungs at the time of weighing. If the volume of air is going to be measured at the time of weighing it does not matter how much air is in the lungs, because it is being measured. The amount of air in the lungs is therefore sometimes called functional residual volume because some, but not all, of the air is expired. Some techniques use a snorkel with a T valve. One side of the T valve is open to the atmosphere; the other is attached to a 5-liter rebreathing bag filled with pure oxygen. The subject submerses and snorkels for several minutes while the water calms. The subject is then instructed to breathe out a "comfortable" amount of air, not all but just some. At that point the valve is closed and the subject cannot breathe for about 20 seconds. At this time his or her actual underwater weight is recorded. After the weight is recorded the T valve is switched to the rebreathing bag of oxygen and the subject is told to breathe and slowly come up from beneath the water. The subject breathes about eight times to equilibrate the air in the lungs with the oxygen in the rebreathing bag. After the subject has taken eight deep breaths the valve on the rebreathing bag is closed, and the "T" is turned to room air. The rebreathing bag is then analyzed for nitrogen and that value is introduced to an equation that results in the volume of the air that was in the lungs at the time of weighing.

Whereas density can be reliably measured, the conversion from density to percent body fat is an estimate. The commonly used calculations are based on assumptions that the density of lean body weight is constant among all people. Several equations are available to estimate percent body fat once the density is determined (see Brozek et al. 1963; Siri 1956). However, Wilmore (1983) warns that the variability of lean-body-weight density can make these equations inappropriate, especially for younger (8- to 12-year-old) and older (72- to 74-year-old) males.

Underwater weighing does not necessarily produce accurate scientific results. The accuracy of the underwater weighing method is a function of the laboratory where it is being done. Many laboratories use an autopsy scale, which, when weighing, fluctuates 2 or 3 lbs, making an accurate weight difficult to obtain. One health club advertised that it did underwater weighing, which was described as the most scientific and most accurate method known. Although the statement about underwater weighing was true, the accuracy of the system was very questionable and could not be compared to a good technique of underwater weighing. The health club used a spring scale with a 10-lb dial, a scuba diver's weight belt, and a tripod frame in the corner of the swimming pool, and the residual volume was estimated at 1500 ml. The degree of precision of the weighing apparatus used can greatly affect the accuracy of underwater weighing. Many systems use a spring-loaded scale for measuring weight underwater. Even with damping, this type of scale does not stabilize during weighing, so the technician must estimate the weight from a moving scale. Load cells or strain gauges with electronic outputs to a printer or plotter record the weight more accurately.

Although percent fat is only an estimate from the density obtained from underwater weighing, it is still the best available estimate. The potential error in underwater weighing of 2.5% is considered minimal. Although it has limitations, underwater weighing is the benchmark for validating other methods.

Skinfold Measurements

When individuals gain fat, much of this added adipose tissue occurs in subcutaneous areas in certain parts of the body. Individuals who gain weight reflect the weight gain in increasing waistlines and larger neck sizes. We tend to put on fat externally. Internal fat also increases but is not as noticeable, and it is not the fat that people, aesthetically, are concerned about. If this excess fat is deposited externally in the subcutaneous areas it can be picked up with the thumb and four fingers; if the skin can be pinched up, then the thickness of the fold can be measured with a caliper. As individuals "put on" weight (fat) these measurements get larger.

Skinfold calipers have been designed to measure the thickness of skin and subcutaneous fat. Good calipers are designed with a constant tension spring, which means that regardless of how wide the caliper jaws spread, the tension between the jaws is constant (see figures 6.1 and 6.2). Jaw pressure differs depending on the different makes of calipers, and care should be taken to use the same caliper when doing "before-and-after" testing. In addition, the same caliper should be used as the caliper that was used to develop the norm tables. The YMCA norm tables were developed using the Lange calipers, so it is recommended that YMCAs use these calipers when assessing members.

Skinfold measurements are excellent estimates of total body fat. Norm tables are included in this book for determining the percentile rank for any particular age and sex and can determine whether an individual is average, below average, or above average in total body fat when compared with other individuals of the same sex and age. Skinfold measurements require only skinfold calipers and skill to be reliable and valid.

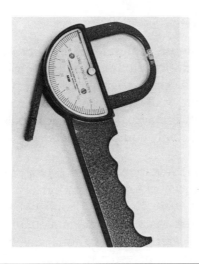

Figure 6.1 Lange skinfold caliper.

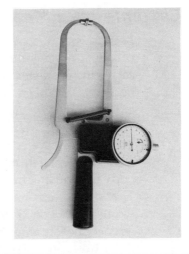

Figure 6.2 Harpenden skinfold caliper.

Considerable practice of skinfold measurements is needed for accuracy, and those who use this method should practice on a group of individuals, recording the measurements until the results become consistent. The same individual may be measured by two different testers to check for consistency, and the difference between the two sets of measurements should not exceed 2 millimeters (mm). If the difference exceeds 2 mm, more practice is needed to standardize the procedure. A coefficient of correlation can be computed on each skinfold location by a simple test-retest procedure of about 20 participants. This procedure was explained earlier.

Skinfold test locations are those sites where fat usually accumulates. Details on sites and measurement techniques are given later in this chapter. The skinfold sites must be exactly the same as those from which the norms were developed. Although many sites can be used, the most commonly used sites are on the chest (pectoral), the abdomen (umbilicus), the hip (ilium or suprailiac), the side (axilla or midaxilla), the posterior upper arm (triceps), the scapula (back or subscapula), and the anterior thigh (quadricep).

The benefits of skinfold measurements are obvious. Little equipment is needed, they can be done quickly, and the interpretation is simple. An individual who has an abdominal skinfold of 28 mm at the start of a program and reduces this measurement to 18 mm in 20 weeks has a reduction of 10 mm in that site's measurement. Skinfold measurements involve no estimate or prediction; they clearly measure the amount of fat in a specific location. Profiles are presented in this chapter that will enable the subject to compare his or her measurement with others of the same sex and age. These profiles also dramatically show the individual where they are "carrying" their fat. It is not uncommon to add the measurements at the various sites and call this amount the total fat. Use caution, however, in comparing total fat measurements to norm tables; be sure that the norm tables use the same sites and the same number of sites.

The major disadvantage of skinfold testing is that too many individuals use the calipers with insufficient practice. Caliper measurements are not reliable when first taken, but they do become very reliable with adequate practice.

Circumference Measurements*

Because skinfold measurements require a high level of expertise resulting from practice and tested reliability, it is difficult to find trained technicians capable of capturing consistent measurements. Alternative methods for predicting percent body fat have been developed using easily measured body circumferences, usually combined with height, weight, and age data. Large numbers of subjects can be measured in a short time, and the only equipment needed is a measuring tape and a weight scale.

McArdle, Katch, and Katch (1981) developed equations for calculating percent body fat by using three circumferences for four population groups: men between 17 and 26 years of age, women between 17 and 26, men between 27 and 50, and women between 27 and 50. From the analysis of the data obtained from circumference measurements and underwater weighing, equations have been developed from which percent body fat can be estimated within 2.5% to 4% of the values obtained by underwater weighing. This range is quite acceptable for most screening purposes.

Although the accuracy of estimating percent body fat by skinfold measurements and circumference measurements is similar, many investigators still prefer skinfolds. Skinfolds measure fat directly, whereas circumferences make no distinction between fat and muscle. Circumference measurements are most accurate when subjects are within an average body-fat range. In an extreme case, using circumference to measure someone with a large amount of muscle mass, such as a bodybuilder, would probably yield an estimated percentage of fat similar to that of an obese person. However, although the obese person might have the same physical size, he or she would have a much greater percentage of body fat than would a bodybuilder.

The anatomical sites selected for measurement vary and may include the circumferences of the abdomen, right thigh, right forearm, right calf, right upper arm, and buttocks. The U.S. Navy is presently using two circumferences to estimate percent body fat—the umbilicus and the neck; both of these measurements have good landmarks and can be taught to people who have little expertise.

Waist Girth and Waist-to-Hip Ratio

Waist girth is a measurement that is familiar to most individuals. It is commonly used for pant and skirt sizes. Most individuals know their waist girth and complain when they gain weight that the waist girth has increased. They are not aware of their percent fat or body composition; all they know is that their clothes are tight, which is reinforced by their increased waist girth. For these reasons it is desirable and of interest to include the waist-girth measurement in any test battery. In addition, a couple of other body composition indices rely on waist girth.

Waist-to-hip ratio (also called abdominal-to-gluteal ratio) is a well used index for risk of disease. Obesity increases the risk of many degenerative diseases, and this index warns individuals when their risk is increasing. The waist girth is divided by the hip girth giving the index. The lower the ratio the less the risk of several debilitating diseases, such as coronary artery disease and diabetes. In men any ratio above 0.9 puts the individual at risk; the higher the ratio, the greater

*Adapted by permission from J. Donahue, L. Golding, and L. Cummings, 1988, "A comparative review of four methods for calculating percent body fat," *Perspective* 14.

the risk. In women any ratio above 0.8 increases the risk of degenerative diseases. An age factor permits a small increase in the ratio with age.

The following is an example using the waist-to-hip ratio: a 40-year-old man has a waist girth of 30 in. and a hip girth of 36 in.; his waist-to-hip ratio is 30/36 = 0.8, which is normal risk. Another 40-year-old man with a larger abdomen (40 in.) and the same hip girth (36 in.) would have a ratio of 1.1, putting him at high risk.

Table 6.1 identifies who is at risk and to what degree they are at risk. In the previous example the first man had a ratio of 0.8. Reading from the table we see that a ratio of 0.8 and an age of 40 years puts this man in the light shaded area or low risk. In the second example the man had a ratio of 1.1; again, reading from the male table we see that a ratio of 1.1 and an age of 40 years puts this individual in the upper white area or very high risk. The women's chart is read in the same manner.

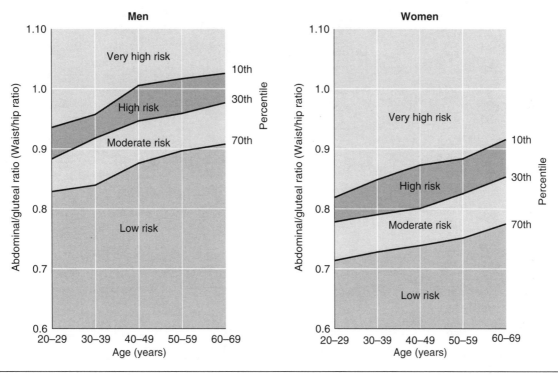

Table 6.1 Degree of risk based on waist-to-hip ratio.

From *Fitness and Sports Medicine,* 3rd ed. by David C. Nieman. Copyright © 1995 by Mayfield Publishing Company. Adapted by permission of the publisher.

Body Mass Index

Because height and weight are commonly measured, another index that has been popular in epidemiological studies is the Body Mass Index (BMI). BMI is obtained by dividing the body weight in kilograms (kg) by the height in meters squared:

$$\frac{\text{Body weight (kg)}}{(\text{Height in meters})^2}$$

Generally speaking, males and females with a BMI of greater than 27 are overweight, and their risk of degenerative disease is increased. Table 6.2 gives the BMI quickly from height and weight without any calculations.

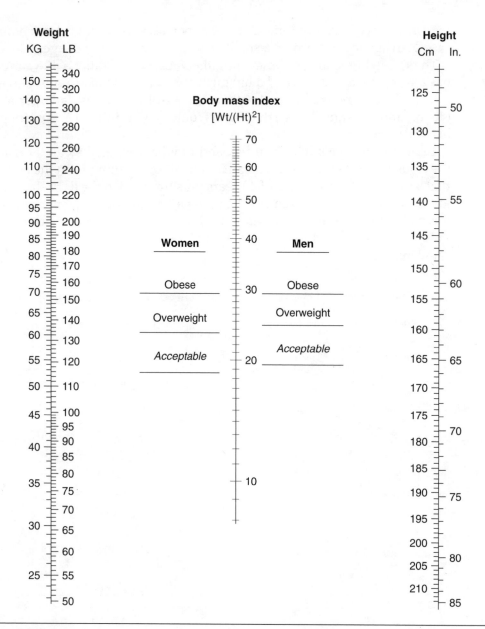

Table 6.2 BMI chart.
Adapted, by permission, from G.A. Bray, 1978, "Definitions, measurements, and classification of the syndrome of obesity," *International Journal of Obesity* 2:99.

The calculations and the interpretations are done through the BMI chart in table 6.3. To read the chart find the height in inches in the left-hand column, then read across to the approximate weight. At the top of that column is the BMI; below the chart, interpretations of the BMI are given in BMI ranges.

Bioelectrical Impedance Analysis (BIA)*

Due in part to a demand for faster and easier methods of evaluating body composition, bioelectrical impedance analysis (BIA) has become a widely used method of estimating percent body fat.

*Adapted by permission from J. Donahue, L. Golding, and L. Cummings, 1988, "A comparative review of four methods for calculating percent body fat," *Perspective* 14.

Table 6.3 Body Mass Index

Height (in)	19	20	21	22	23	24	25	26	27	28	29	30	35	40
						Weight (lbs)								
58	91	96	100	105	110	115	119	124	129	134	138	143	167	191
59	94	99	104	109	114	119	124	128	133	138	143	148	173	198
60	97	102	107	112	118	123	128	133	138	143	148	153	179	204
61	100	106	111	116	122	127	132	137	143	148	153	158	185	211
62	104	109	115	120	126	131	136	142	147	153	158	164	191	218
63	107	113	118	124	130	135	141	146	152	158	163	169	197	225
64	110	116	122	128	134	140	145	151	157	163	169	174	204	232
65	114	120	126	132	138	144	150	156	162	168	174	180	210	240
66	118	124	130	136	142	148	155	161	167	173	179	186	216	247
67	121	127	134	140	146	153	159	166	172	178	185	191	223	255
68	125	131	138	144	151	158	164	171	177	184	190	197	230	262
69	128	135	142	149	155	162	169	176	182	189	196	203	236	270
70	132	139	146	153	160	167	174	181	188	195	202	207	243	278
71	136	143	150	157	165	172	179	186	193	200	208	215	250	286
72	140	147	154	162	169	177	184	191	199	206	213	221	258	294
73	144	151	159	166	174	182	189	197	204	212	219	227	265	302
74	148	155	163	171	179	186	194	202	210	218	225	233	272	311
75	152	160	168	176	184	192	200	208	216	224	232	240	279	319
76	156	164	172	180	189	197	205	213	221	230	238	246	287	328

Less than 20 Weight gain may be advisable	20-25 Acceptable range for most people but potential health problems with weight gain	26-27 Escalating health risks	Higher than 27 Dramatic risk of health problems

The use of BIA is based on the principle that the conductivity of an electrical impulse is greater through fat-free tissue than it is through fatty tissue. Through electrodes on the hand and foot, the instrument measures a small electrical current passing between the electrodes and therefore the body's impedance (resistance) to the electrical current. Depending on whether there is more fatty or fat-free tissue, the flow of the current will be different. The analyzer measures the flow and *estimates* the amount of fatty tissue in the body. Impedance is measured in ohms. The ohmmeter interfaces with a computer that calculates body density using a series of algebraic equations (a constant multiplies by the weight, and the resistance is divided by the square of the height). The result of the impedance determines total body water. The total body water is then introduced into an equation to estimate density, and an equation is used to convert density to percent body fat.

Once it has the figure obtained for percent body fat, the BIA computer provides printouts for a variety of information specific to each individual, including the percent and absolute amount of body fat, total body water, and lean body weight. Optional printouts can include nutrition tables, diet and exercise programs, energy expenditure charts, and suggested weight-loss or weight-gain charts.

The attractiveness and marketability of BIA are its speed (about 5 minutes per subject), ease of operation, and self-explanatory computer printouts. Participant compliance with suggestions to improve health is boosted by the "printout mystique," the belief that computers are infallible. The provider's image may also benefit by association with this visible high-tech equipment.

The output of a computer, however, is no more accurate than its input. In the case of BIA, if the assumptions and formulas used in the computer program are not valid, many of the parameters printed out may have a poor relationship to what was measured. The validity and reliability of BIA continues to be studied. The first research on this method largely documented the shortcomings of BIA. McArdle et al. (1981) found an overestimation of body fat using BIA in absolute terms of 6.8% for young males. Scientific papers presented at the 1985 annual meeting of the American College of Sports Medicine showed both overestimations and underestimations of percent body fat for various populations. In most of these studies the body-fat estimations were calculated using the software supplied by the manufacturer of BIA instruments. Lohman conducted a study using seven research centers to develop better formulae specific to different populations for estimations of percent body fat using BIA. Although BIA measurements today are infinitely better than when they were first introduced and results show a better relationship with underwater weighing, research has yet to prove conclusively the reliability of this type of body composition measurement.

In 1994 the National Institutes of Health published a statement titled "Bioelectrical Impedance Analysis in Body Composition Measurement." National experts in the field, including scientists from nutrition, pediatrics, surgery, public health, biomedical engineering, epidemiology, and physiology reviewed all available research in developing the statement. Here are their conclusions:

> *"BIA values are affected by numerous variables including body position, hydration status, consumption of food and beverages, ambient air and skin temperature, recent physical activity, and conductance of the examining table. Reliable BIA requires standardization and control of these variables."*

> *"The ability of BIA to accurately predict adiposity in severely obese individuals is limited. In addition, BIA is not useful in measuring short-term changes in body composition (i.e., in response to diet or exercise) among individuals."*

> *"Available information indicates that BIA is not useful in measuring acute changes in body fat in individuals."*

> *"BIA technology does not provide information on regional distribution or patterning of body fat."*

> *"A specific, well-defined procedure for performing routine BIA measurements is not practiced. Therefore, the NIH recommends the setting of instrument standards and procedural methods."*

Although BIA can be reasonably reliable with proper equipment, procedures, and interpretation of results, the control of these variables in settings such as YMCAs may not always be consistent. BIA appears to fall within the same range of accuracy as other methods of estimating body composition, such as infrared technology and BMI. YMCAs should consider the relative cost of BIA compared to the recommended method of skinfold measurements.

Near-Infrared

Near-infrared technology is another technique for estimating percent body fat. The technique involves a wand with an infrared source. This wand is placed on the anterior biceps, and the infrared beam is introduced. The infrared is reflected off the underlying tissue; the estimate of fatty tissue determined by the infrared beam is correlated to underwater weighing. To date, little scientific documentation indicates that infrared is a valid method.

Prediction Equations

Prediction equations are statistical procedures for estimating body composition from simple anthropometrical measurements. The results are validated by comparison to hydrostatic weighing.

The research literature includes several prediction equations, and many have proven to be highly reliable and valid. Because the measurements used in these equations are taken on specific populations, they are usually accurate only when applied to a similar population. Therefore, different equations have been published for young boys, young recruits in the army, adult males, high school girls, and adult women. The measurements taken may be skinfolds, circumferences, bone diameters, or any other anthropometrical measurement. These equations are computer generated when compared to density obtained through underwater weighing. The measurements used in the equations are usually simple to take, making equations an easy field technique. Because these equations are population specific, several different equations need to be used on different groups of people (e.g., men, women, young, old).

Jackson and Pollock (1978) published an equation based on measurements from 403 adult men between the ages of 18 and 61. They found that a limitation on many of the previously published equations was that the slopes of the regression lines for the various groups were not parallel. This difference resulted in biased body-density estimates. Their studies have shown that the relationship between skinfold measurements and body density is not linear but rather curvilinear.

The Jackson-Pollock study divided 403 subjects into a validation group of 308 and a cross-validation group of 95. Body density was determined by hydrostatic weighing. Regression analysis was used to derive the generalized equation. Polynomial models were used to test whether the relationship between body density and the sum of skinfolds was curvilinear. The authors found that the relationship between skinfold fat and body density was quadratic. Age was used as an independent variable and eliminated the need for several age-adjusted equations. The authors conducted a study of women, which resulted in the development of equations that exhibited similar statistical characteristics. A further discussion of this equation is found in the section on estimating percent body fat.

The Jackson and Pollock equation based on seven skinfold sites was published in the *British Journal of Nutrition*. When earlier versions of the *Y's Way to Physical Fitness* were being written, Jackson and Pollock were both on the team of people writing the book, and they developed, from their data, two equations especially for the YMCA. These equations used the sum of four skinfold sites (the abdomen, ilium, triceps, and thigh). Because the thigh measurement is occasionally difficult to take, Jackson and Pollock developed a second equation based on the sum of three skinfold sites (abdomen, ilium, and triceps). These two equations are still used in the YMCA Fitness Assessment protocol.

Percent Body Fat and Target Weight

All but one of the preceding procedures result in the estimation of percent body fat. If the percent body fat is known, a desirable weight can be determined. Desirable weight is called *target weight*. Target weight is *lean body weight* (the body weight with no fat) plus some desired percentage of fat. Target weight is a better term than ideal weight. It is the weight that an individual is aiming to attain. Ideal weight brings up the question of "ideal for whom?" Is the weight ideal for a marathoner, ideal for a linebacker, ideal for a gymnast, etc.? The desired weight for different groups changes. Marathon runners may wish to be 10% to 12% fat (as many marathon runners are), whereas weight lifters or football players may prefer to be 19% to 20% fat.

It has been suggested that from a health standpoint adult men should be 16% fat. This number may be a little low for the average male. Men should, however, be under 20% fat and, from an aesthetic and training standpoint, be 16% fat or less. The YMCA uses the range of 16% to 20% as their range for normal. When YMCA fitness specialists calculate a male's target weight they determine it at 16%. Adult women should be between 19% and 23% fat. Many women find, however, that 19% body fat is difficult to obtain; the YMCA determines the target weight for women at 23%. Women should be 23% fat or less. Although standards may differ from one laboratory to another, a man with over 25% fat and a woman with over 35% fat would certainly be considered to have marginal obesity. The new norms collected on 35,000 individuals show that men (depending on their age) average between 13% and 25% body fat; women average between 22% and 32%.

Individuals who are obese should be warned of the potential health hazards of obesity and the desirability of bringing one's weight within a more normal range. The fitness director could recommend, in consultation with a physician, a program of diet and exercise that would produce a gradual weight loss. Crash diets are unwise from a health standpoint and are rarely successful in keeping weight off. A realistic goal is a caloric deficit, obtained through a diet and exercise regimen, of no more than 500 kcal per day, continuing until the desired weight is achieved. It should be remembered in recommending exercise for an overweight individual that practically all work is more difficult due to the excess weight, and consideration must be given to the type and intensity of exercise that can be tolerated by this person.

The computation of target weight is accomplished after the determination of percent fat. The method described later in this chapter results in a percent fat for a certain age. After this percentage is determined, a target weight is computed as follows:

Example 1. Subject A: male, 40 years old, weighs 210 lb. He is 23% fat as determined by the Jackson-Pollock equation (or by any other method).

a. If 23% of his weight is fat, his fat weight in pounds is determined by calculating 23% of his total weight (23% of 210 lb = 48.3 lb of fat).

b. Based on the two-compartment model mentioned earlier in this chapter, subtracting the fat weight (one compartment) from the total weight will result in a number for the other compartment (lean body weight). Therefore in this example subtracting his fat weight (48.3 lb) from his total weight (210 lb) will give his lean body weight (LBW): 210 − 48.3 = 161.7. Without fat his body weight is 161.7 lb.

c. Instead of 23% fat, he should be 16% fat. His weight at 16% is obtained by taking his LBW (161.7) and adding 16% fat: LBW/0.84 = weight at 16% fat, or 161.7/0.84 = 192.5 lb (100% − 16% = 0.84.)

Table 6.4 allows this figure to be determined without computation. Actual weight (210) is found along the top of the table, percent fat (23%) is found along the left-hand side, and the point where these two columns intersect is the target weight (193 lb at 16%). (This result is 192.5 lb if computed as just shown in the prior example.)

Example 2. Subject B: female, 35 years old, weight 145 lb. She is 28% fat as determined by the Jackson-Pollock equation.

a. If 28% of her weight is fat, her fat weight in pounds is determined by calculating 28% of her total weight (28% of 145 lb = 40.6 lb of fat).

b. Subtracting this fat weight from her total weight will give her LBW: 145 − 40.6 = 104.4 lb. Without fat her body weight is 104.4 lb.

c. Instead of 28% fat she should be 23% fat. This target fat percentage is obtained as above by dividing her LBW by the desired percentage subtracted from 100%. Thus LBW/0.77 gives the desired weight at 23% fat, or 104.4/0.77 = 135.6 lb. (0.77 is 100% minus 23%.) Table 6.5 gives recommended target weights for women.

Table 6.4 Target Weight—Men (16% Fat)

% fat	Body weight (lb)																								
	120	125	130	135	140	145	150	155	160	165	170	175	180	185	190	195	200	205	210	215	220	225	230	235	240
17	119	123	129	133	138	143	148	153	158	163	168	173	179	183	188	193	198	203	208	212	217	222	227	232	237
18	117	122	127	132	137	142	146	151	156	161	166	171	176	181	186	190	195	200	205	210	215	220	225	229	234
19	116	121	125	130	135	140	145	149	154	159	164	169	174	178	183	188	193	198	203	207	212	217	222	225	231
20	114	119	124	129	133	138	143	148	152	157	162	167	171	176	181	186	190	195	200	205	210	214	219	224	229
21	113	118	122	127	132	136	141	146	150	155	160	165	169	174	179	183	188	193	198	202	207	212	216	221	226
22	111	116	121	125	130	135	139	144	149	153	158	162	167	172	176	181	186	190	195	200	204	209	214	218	223
23	110	115	119	123	128	133	138	142	147	151	156	160	165	170	174	179	183	188	193	197	202	206	211	215	220
24	109	113	118	122	127	131	136	140	145	149	154	158	163	167	172	176	181	186	190	195	199	204	208	213	217
25	107	112	116	121	125	129	134	138	143	147	152	156	161	165	170	174	179	183	188	192	196	201	205	210	214
26	106	110	115	119	123	128	132	137	141	145	150	154	159	163	167	172	176	181	185	189	194	198	203	207	211
27	104	109	113	117	122	126	130	135	139	143	148	152	156	161	165	169	174	178	183	187	191	196	200	204	209
28	103	107	111	116	120	124	129	133	137	141	146	150	154	159	163	167	171	176	180	184	189	193	197	201	208
29	101	106	110	114	118	123	127	131	135	139	144	148	152	156	161	165	169	173	178	182	186	190	194	199	203
30	100	104	108	113	117	121	125	129	133	137	142	146	150	154	158	162	167	171	175	179	183	188	192	196	200
31	99	103	107	111	115	119	123	127	131	136	140	144	149	152	156	160	164	168	173	177	181	185	189	193	197
32	97	101	105	109	113	117	121	125	130	134	138	142	146	150	154	158	162	166	170	174	178	182	186	190	194
33	96	100	104	108	112	116	120	124	128	132	136	140	144	148	152	156	160	164	168	171	175	179	183	187	191
34	94	98	102	106	110	114	118	122	126	130	134	137	141	145	149	153	157	161	165	169	173	177	181	185	189
35	93	97	101	104	108	112	116	120	124	128	132	135	139	143	147	151	155	159	163	166	170	174	178	182	186
36	91	95	99	103	107	110	114	118	122	126	130	133	137	141	145	149	152	156	160	164	168	171	175	179	183
37	90	94	98	101	105	109	113	116	120	124	128	131	135	139	143	146	150	154	158	161	165	169	173	176	180
38	89	92	96	100	103	107	111	114	118	122	125	129	133	137	140	144	148	151	155	159	162	166	170	174	177
39	87	91	94	98	102	105	109	112	116	120	123	127	131	134	138	142	145	149	153	156	160	163	167	171	174
40	86	89	93	96	100	104	107	111	114	118	121	125	129	132	136	139	143	146	150	154	157	161	164	168	173

Note. To use, find the subject's present weight at the top of the table, then descend vertically to the horizontal row corresponding to the estimated percent fat. For example, the target weight for a man who weighed 210 lb and was 23% fat would be 193 lb (see text for computation).

Occasionally a person will be measured whose percent body fat is lower than the norm. This has sometimes caused concern in interpretation. For example, if a male subject is 12% body fat as determined by the Jackson-Pollock equation and weighs 167 lb, his weight should not be interpreted as a need to gain 4% body fat. The target weight is based on the general population. This individual should be told that he is in the range of very fit marathon runners and that it is often desirable to be under the norm; most athletes are. Because the target weight is based on the general population, however, tables 6.4 and 6.5 do not go under 17% and 24%, respectively.

Estimation of Body Fat by Skinfolds

The YMCA method of estimating body fat involves the measurement of skinfolds in various body locations. The body composition test of the YMCA Fitness Assessment protocol has three components:

1. The seven actual skinfolds are put on the body composition profile for each age and sex.

2. Four of those skinfolds are used in the Jackson-Pollock sum-of-four equation, resulting in percent body fat.

3. Target weight is determined from the percent body fat.

To estimate percent body fat, the YMCA uses the Jackson-Pollock sum-of-four equation. It is not necessary for the fitness tester to know the actual equation, but it is presented in figure 6.3 (on page 125) for those who are interested. Tables based on the sums of skinfold measurements and on age are included in this chapter to allow direct readings of percent body fat and target weight without the need to perform any calculations (see tables 6.6 and 6.7).

Both men and women use the sum of four sites: the abdomen, ilium, triceps, and thigh. As mentioned earlier, experience has shown that accurate measurement of the thigh is sometimes difficult, so Jackson and Pollock constructed additional tables that eliminate the thigh measurement. The equations based on the sum of three sites (abdomen, ilium, and triceps) should be used only if the thigh skinfold cannot be measured accurately.

The fitness director should attempt to measure the four skinfold sites and use tables 6.6 and 6.7 to estimate percent fat for men and women, respectively. If the thigh measurement cannot be taken or appears inaccurate, then the sum of three sites should be used. Two examples of finding the target weight with four skinfold site measurements follow.

Example 1. Subject A: male, 40 years old, 210 lb
Skinfold Measurements

Abdomen	31 mm
Ilium	26 mm
Triceps	14 mm
Thigh	21 mm
Sum of 4	92 mm

Table 6.5 Target Weight—Women (23% Fat)

% fat	Body weight (lb)																		
	105	110	115	120	125	130	135	140	145	150	155	160	165	170	175	180	185	190	195
24	104	109	114	118	123	128	133	138	143	148	153	158	163	168	173	178	183	188	192
25	102	107	112	117	122	127	131	136	141	146	151	156	161	166	170	175	180	185	190
26	101	106	111	115	120	125	130	135	139	144	149	154	159	163	168	173	178	183	187
27	100	104	109	114	119	123	128	133	137	142	147	152	156	161	166	171	175	180	185
28	98	103	108	112	117	122	126	131	136	140	145	150	154	159	163	168	173	178	182
29	97	101	106	111	115	120	124	129	134	138	143	148	152	157	161	166	171	175	180
30	95	100	105	109	114	118	123	127	132	136	141	145	150	155	159	164	168	173	177
31	94	99	103	108	112	116	121	125	130	134	139	144	148	152	157	161	166	170	175
32	93	97	102	106	110	115	119	124	129	132	137	141	146	150	155	159	163	168	172
33	91	96	100	104	109	113	117	122	126	131	135	139	144	148	152	157	161	165	170
34	90	94	99	103	107	111	116	120	124	129	133	137	141	146	150	154	159	163	167
35	89	93	97	101	106	110	114	118	122	127	131	135	139	144	148	152	156	160	165
36	87	91	96	100	104	108	112	116	121	125	129	133	137	141	145	150	154	158	162
37	86	90	94	98	102	106	110	115	119	123	127	131	135	139	143	147	151	155	160
38	85	89	93	97	101	105	109	113	117	121	125	129	133	137	141	145	149	153	157
39	83	87	91	95	99	103	107	111	115	119	123	127	131	135	139	143	147	151	154
40	82	86	90	94	97	101	105	109	113	117	121	125	129	132	136	140	144	148	152

Note. To use, find the subject's present weight at the top of the table, then descend vertically to the horizontal row corresponding to the estimated percent fat. For example, the target weight for a woman who weighed 145 lb and was 28% fat would be 136 lb (see text for computation.)

Four Sites

Percent Fat: Men

Sum of four sites:

1. Abdomen
2. Ilium
3. Tricep
4. Thigh

Percent fat = .29288 ($\Sigma 4$) − .0005 ($\Sigma 4^2$) + .15845 (AGE) − 5.76377

$R = .901$ $\qquad\qquad$ $SE = 3.49\%$ fat

Percent Fat: Women

Sum of four sites:

1. Abdomen
2. Ilium
3. Tricep
4. Thigh

Percent fat = .29669 ($\Sigma 4$) − .00043 ($\Sigma 4^2$) + .02963 (AGE) + 1.4072

$R = .846$ $\qquad\qquad$ $SE = 3.89\%$ fat

Three Sites

Percent Fat: Men

Sum of three sites:

1. Abdomen
2. Ilium
3. Tricep

Percent fat = .39287 ($\Sigma 3$) − .00105 ($\Sigma 3^2$) + .15772 (AGE) − 5.18845

$R = .893$ $\qquad\qquad$ $SE = 3.63\%$ fat

Percent Fat: Women

Sum of three sites:

1. Abdomen
2. Ilium
3. Tricep

Percent fat = .41563 ($\Sigma 3$) − .00112 ($\Sigma 3^2$) + .03661 (AGE) + 4.03653

$R = .825$ $\qquad\qquad$ $SE = 3.98\%$ fat

Figure 6.3 The Jackson-Pollock equations for four sites and three sites.

Table 6.6 Percent Fat Estimates for Four Sites—Men

Sum of 4 skinfolds	Age to last year								
	18-22	23-27	28-32	33-37	38-42	43-47	48-52	53-57	58
13-17	1.7	2.5	3.3	4.1	4.9	5.6	6.4	7.2	8.0
18-22	3.1	3.9	4.6	5.4	6.2	7.0	7.8	8.6	9.4
23-27	4.4	5.2	6.0	6.8	7.6	8.4	9.2	10.0	10.7
28-32	5.7	6.5	7.3	8.1	8.9	9.7	10.5	11.3	12.1
33-37	7.0	7.8	8.6	9.4	10.2	11.0	11.8	12.6	13.4
38-42	8.3	9.1	9.9	10.7	11.5	12.3	13.1	13.9	14.6
43-47	9.6	10.3	11.1	11.9	12.7	13.5	14.3	15.1	15.9
48-52	10.8	11.6	12.4	13.2	13.9	14.7	15.5	16.3	17.1
53-57	12.0	12.8	13.6	14.4	15.1	15.9	16.7	17.5	18.3
58-62	13.1	13.9	14.7	15.5	16.3	17.1	17.9	18.7	19.5
63-67	14.3	15.1	15.9	16.7	17.5	18.2	19.0	19.8	20.6
68-72	15.4	16.2	17.0	17.8	18.6	19.4	20.2	21.0	21.8
73-77	16.5	17.3	18.1	18.9	19.7	20.5	21.3	22.1	22.8
78-82	17.6	18.4	19.2	20.0	20.7	21.5	22.3	23.1	23.9
83-87	18.6	19.4	20.2	21.0	21.8	22.6	23.4	24.2	25.0
88-92	19.6	20.4	21.2	22.0	22.8	23.6	24.4	25.2	26.0
93-97	20.6	21.4	22.2	23.0	23.8	24.6	25.4	26.2	27.0
98-102	21.6	22.4	23.2	24.0	24.8	25.6	26.4	27.1	27.9
103-107	22.5	23.3	24.1	24.9	25.7	26.5	27.3	28.1	28.9
108-112	23.5	24.2	25.0	25.8	26.6	27.4	28.2	29.0	29.8
113-117	24.3	25.1	25.9	26.7	27.5	28.3	29.1	29.9	30.7
118-122	25.2	26.0	26.8	27.6	28.4	29.2	30.0	30.8	31.6
123-127	26.0	26.8	27.6	28.4	29.2	30.0	30.8	31.6	32.4
128-132	26.9	27.7	28.4	29.2	30.0	30.8	31.6	32.4	33.2
133-137	27.7	28.4	29.2	30.0	30.8	31.6	32.4	33.2	34.0
138-142	28.4	29.2	30.0	30.8	31.6	32.4	33.2	34.0	34.8
143-147	29.2	29.9	30.7	31.5	32.3	33.1	33.9	34.7	35.5
148-152	29.9	30.7	31.5	32.2	33.0	33.8	34.6	35.4	36.2
153-157	30.6	31.3	32.1	32.9	33.7	34.5	35.3	36.1	36.9
158-162	31.2	32.0	32.8	33.6	34.4	35.2	36.0	36.8	37.6
163-167	31.8	32.6	33.4	34.2	35.0	35.8	36.6	37.4	38.2
168-172	32.5	33.3	34.0	34.8	35.6	36.4	37.2	38.0	38.8
173-177	33.0	33.8	34.6	35.4	36.2	37.0	37.8	38.6	39.4
178-182	33.6	34.4	35.2	36.0	36.8	37.6	38.4	39.2	39.9
183-187	34.1	34.9	35.7	36.5	37.3	38.1	38.9	39.7	40.5

Table 6.7 Percent Fat Estimates for Four Sites—Women

Sum of 4 skinfolds	Age to last year								
	18-22	23-27	28-32	33-37	38-42	43-47	48-52	53-57	58
23-27	8.6	9.3	9.4	9.6	9.7	9.9	10.0	10.2	10.3
28-32	10.0	10.7	10.8	11.0	11.0	11.3	11.4	11.6	11.7
33-37	11.3	12.0	12.2	12.3	12.4	12.6	12.7	12.9	13.0
38-42	12.6	13.3	13.5	13.6	13.7	13.9	14.1	14.2	14.4
43-47	13.9	14.6	14.8	14.9	15.0	15.2	15.4	15.5	15.7
48-52	15.2	15.9	16.1	16.2	16.3	16.5	16.7	16.8	17.0
53-57	16.5	17.2	17.3	17.5	17.5	17.8	17.9	18.1	18.2
58-62	17.7	18.4	18.6	18.7	18.8	19.0	19.1	19.3	19.4
63-67	18.9	19.6	19.8	19.9	20.0	20.2	20.4	20.5	20.7
68-72	20.1	20.8	21.0	21.1	21.2	21.4	21.6	21.7	21.9
73-77	21.3	22.0	22.1	22.3	22.3	22.6	22.7	22.9	23.0
78-82	22.5	23.1	23.3	23.4	23.5	23.7	23.9	24.0	24.2
83-87	23.6	24.3	24.4	24.6	24.6	24.9	25.0	25.2	25.3
88-92	24.7	25.4	25.5	25.7	25.7	26.0	26.1	26.3	26.4
93-97	25.8	26.5	26.6	26.8	26.8	27.1	27.2	27.4	27.5
98-102	26.8	27.5	27.7	27.8	27.9	28.1	28.3	28.4	28.6
103-107	27.9	28.6	28.7	28.9	28.9	29.2	29.3	29.5	29.6
108-112	28.9	29.6	29.7	29.9	30.0	30.2	30.3	30.5	30.6
113-117	29.9	30.6	30.7	30.9	31.0	31.2	31.3	31.5	31.6
118-122	30.9	31.6	31.7	31.9	31.9	32.2	32.3	32.5	32.6
123-127	31.9	32.5	32.7	32.8	32.9	33.1	33.3	33.4	33.6
128-132	32.8	33.5	33.6	33.8	33.8	34.1	34.2	34.4	34.5
133-137	33.7	34.4	34.5	34.7	34.7	35.0	35.1	35.3	35.4
138-142	34.6	35.3	35.4	35.6	35.6	35.9	36.0	36.2	36.3
143-147	35.5	36.2	36.3	36.5	36.5	36.7	36.9	37.0	37.2
148-152	36.3	37.0	37.2	37.3	37.4	37.6	37.8	37.9	38.0
153-157	37.2	37.8	38.0	38.1	38.2	38.4	38.6	38.7	38.9
158-162	38.0	38.6	38.8	38.9	39.0	39.2	39.4	39.5	39.7
163-167	38.8	39.4	39.6	39.7	39.8	40.0	40.2	40.3	40.5
168-172	39.5	40.2	40.3	40.5	40.6	40.8	40.9	41.1	41.2
173-177	40.3	40.9	41.1	41.2	41.3	41.5	41.7	41.8	42.0
178-182	41.0	41.7	41.8	42.0	42.0	42.3	42.4	42.6	42.7
183-187	41.7	42.4	42.5	42.7	42.7	43.0	43.1	43.3	43.4
188-192	42.4	43.0	43.2	43.3	43.4	43.6	43.8	43.9	44.1
193-197	43.0	43.7	43.9	44.0	44.1	44.3	44.4	44.6	44.7
198-202	43.7	44.3	44.5	44.6	44.7	44.9	45.1	45.2	45.4

Using table 6.6, which presents the sums of four skinfolds for men, a total of 92 mm and an age of 40 at the last birthday yields a percentage of fat of 22.8. To find the target weight, turn to table 6.4. Reading across from the left-hand column under percent body fat to the body weight column of 210 lb, we find that Subject A has a target weight of 193 lb.

Example 2. Subject B: female, 35 years old, 145 lb
Skinfold Measurements

Abdomen	28 mm
Ilium	23 mm
Triceps	18 mm
Thigh	33 mm
Sum of 4	102 mm

Using table 6.7, which presents the sums of four skinfolds for women, a total of 102 mm and an age of 35 at the last birthday yields a percentage of fat of 27.8. To find the target weight, turn to table 6.5 and read across. Subject B has a target weight of 136 lb.

If you cannot use the sum of four because the thigh measurement cannot be taken, you must rely on tables 6.8 and 6.9. The next two examples illustrate finding the target weight using three skinfold sites.

Example 3. Subject A: male, 40 years old, 210 lb
Skinfold Measurements

Abdomen	31 mm
Ilium	26 mm
Triceps	14 mm
Sum of 3	71 mm

Using table 6.8, which presents the sums of three skinfolds for men, a total of 71 mm and an age of 40 at the last birthday yields a percentage of fat of 23.5. To find the target weight, turn to table 6.4. Subject A has a target weight of 191 lb.

Example 4. Subject B: female, 35 years old, 145 lb
Skinfold Measurements

Abdomen	28 mm
Ilium	23 mm
Triceps	18 mm
Sum of 3	69 mm

Using table 6.9, which presents the sums of three skinfolds for women, a total of 69 mm and an age of 35 at the last birthday yields a percentage of fat of 28.9. To find the target weight, turn to table 6.5. Subject B has a target weight of 134 lb.

Table 6.8 Percent Fat Estimates for Three Sites—Men

Sum of 3 skinfolds	Age to last year								
	18-22	23-27	28-32	33-37	38-42	43-47	48-52	53-57	58
8-12	1.8	2.6	3.4	4.2	4.9	5.7	6.5	7.3	8.1
13-17	3.6	4.4	5.2	6.0	6.8	7.6	8.4	9.1	9.9
18-22	5.4	6.2	7.0	7.8	8.6	9.3	10.1	10.9	11.7
23-27	7.1	7.9	8.7	9.5	10.3	11.1	11.9	12.6	13.4
28-32	8.8	9.6	10.4	11.2	12.0	12.8	13.5	14.3	15.1
33-37	10.4	11.2	12.0	12.8	13.6	14.4	15.2	15.9	16.7
38-42	12.0	12.8	13.6	14.4	15.2	15.9	16.7	17.5	18.3
43-47	13.5	14.3	15.1	15.9	16.7	17.5	18.3	19.0	19.8
48-52	15.0	15.8	16.6	17.4	18.1	18.9	19.7	20.5	21.3
53-57	16.4	17.2	18.0	18.8	19.6	20.3	21.1	21.9	22.7
58-62	17.8	18.5	19.3	20.1	20.9	21.7	22.5	23.3	24.1
63-67	19.1	19.9	20.6	21.4	22.2	23.0	23.8	24.6	25.4
68-72	20.3	21.1	21.9	22.7	23.5	24.3	25.1	25.8	26.6
73-77	21.5	22.3	23.1	23.9	24.7	25.5	26.3	27.0	27.8
78-82	22.7	23.5	24.3	25.0	25.8	26.6	27.4	28.2	29.0
83-87	23.8	24.6	25.3	26.1	26.9	27.7	28.5	29.3	30.1
88-92	24.8	25.6	26.4	27.2	28.0	28.8	29.6	30.3	31.1
93-97	25.8	26.6	27.4	28.2	29.0	29.8	30.5	31.3	32.1
98-102	26.7	27.5	28.3	29.1	29.9	30.7	31.5	32.3	33.1
103-107	27.6	28.4	29.2	30.0	30.8	31.6	32.4	33.2	33.9
108-112	28.5	29.3	30.1	30.8	31.6	32.4	33.2	34.0	34.8
113-117	29.3	30.0	30.8	31.6	32.4	33.2	34.0	34.8	35.6
118-122	30.0	30.8	31.6	32.4	33.1	33.9	34.7	35.5	36.3
123-127	30.7	31.5	32.2	33.0	33.8	34.6	35.4	36.2	37.0
128-132	31.3	32.1	32.9	33.7	34.4	35.2	36.0	36.8	37.6
133-137	31.9	32.7	33.4	34.2	35.0	35.8	36.6	37.4	38.2
138-142	32.4	33.2	34.0	34.8	35.5	36.3	37.1	37.9	38.7
143-147	32.9	33.6	34.4	35.2	36.0	36.8	37.6	38.4	39.2
148-152	33.3	34.1	34.8	35.6	36.4	37.2	38.0	38.8	39.6
153-157	33.6	34.4	35.2	36.0	36.8	37.6	38.4	39.2	39.9
158-162	33.9	34.7	35.5	36.3	37.1	37.9	38.7	39.5	40.3
163-167	34.2	35.0	35.8	36.6	37.4	38.1	38.9	39.7	40.5
168-172	34.4	35.2	36.0	36.8	37.6	38.4	39.1	39.9	40.7
173-177	34.6	35.3	36.1	36.9	37.7	38.5	39.3	40.1	40.9
178-182	34.7	35.4	36.2	37.0	37.8	38.6	39.4	40.2	41.0

Table 6.9 Percent Fat Estimates for Three Sites—Women

Sum of 3 skinfolds	Age to last year								
	18-22	23-27	28-32	33-37	38-42	43-47	48-52	53-57	58
8-12	8.8	9.0	9.2	9.4	9.5	9.7	9.9	10.1	10.3
13-17	10.8	10.9	11.1	11.3	11.5	11.7	11.8	12.0	12.2
18-22	12.6	12.8	13.0	13.2	13.4	13.5	13.7	13.9	14.1
23-27	14.5	14.6	14.8	15.0	15.2	15.4	15.6	15.7	15.9
28-32	16.2	16.4	16.6	16.8	17.0	17.1	17.3	17.5	17.7
33-37	17.9	18.1	18.3	18.5	18.7	18.9	19.0	19.2	19.4
38-42	19.6	19.8	20.0	20.2	20.3	20.5	20.7	20.9	21.1
43-47	21.2	21.4	21.6	21.8	21.9	22.1	22.3	22.5	22.7
48-52	22.8	22.9	23.1	23.3	23.5	23.7	23.8	24.0	24.2
53-57	24.2	24.4	24.6	24.8	25.0	25.2	25.3	25.5	25.7
58-62	25.7	25.9	26.0	26.2	26.4	26.6	26.8	27.0	27.1
63-67	27.1	27.2	27.4	27.6	27.8	28.0	28.2	28.3	28.5
68-72	28.4	28.6	28.7	28.9	29.1	29.3	29.5	29.7	29.8
73-77	29.6	29.8	30.0	30.2	30.4	30.6	30.7	30.9	31.1
78-82	30.9	31.0	31.2	31.4	31.6	31.8	31.9	32.1	32.3
83-87	32.0	32.2	32.4	32.6	32.7	32.9	33.1	33.3	33.5
88-92	33.1	33.3	33.5	33.7	33.8	34.0	34.2	34.4	34.6
93-97	34.1	34.3	34.5	34.7	34.9	35.1	35.2	35.4	35.6
98-102	35.1	35.3	35.5	35.7	35.9	36.0	36.2	36.4	36.6
103-107	36.1	36.2	36.4	36.6	36.8	37.0	37.2	37.3	37.5
108-112	36.9	37.1	37.3	37.5	37.7	37.9	38.0	38.2	38.4
113-117	37.8	37.9	38.1	38.3	39.2	39.4	39.6	39.8	39.5
118-122	38.5	38.7	38.9	39.1	39.4	39.6	39.8	40.0	40.0
123-127	39.2	39.4	39.6	39.8	40.0	40.1	40.3	40.5	40.7
128-132	39.9	40.1	40.2	40.4	40.6	40.8	41.0	41.2	41.3
133-137	40.5	40.7	40.8	41.0	41.2	41.4	41.6	41.7	41.9
138-142	41.0	41.2	41.4	41.6	41.7	41.9	42.1	42.3	42.5
143-147	41.5	41.7	41.9	42.0	42.2	42.4	42.6	42.8	43.0
148-152	41.9	42.1	42.3	42.8	42.6	42.8	43.0	43.2	43.4
153-157	42.3	42.5	42.6	52.8	43.0	43.2	43.4	43.6	43.7
158-162	42.6	42.8	43.0	43.1	43.3	43.5	43.7	43.9	44.1
163-167	42.9	43.0	43.2	43.4	43.6	43.8	44.0	44.1	44.3
168-172	43.1	43.2	43.4	43.6	43.8	44.0	44.2	44.3	44.5
173-177	43.2	43.4	43.6	43.8	43.9	44.1	44.3	44.5	44.7
178-182	43.3	43.5	43.7	43.8	44.0	44.2	44.4	44.6	44.8

Skinfold Measurements Technique

The skinfold measurements are used to determine the percent body fat as just described. The skinfold measurements as raw scores are also valuable and should supplement the information on percent body fat and target weight. Very often a participant in an exercise program reduces the subcutaneous fat in a number of locations, and these individual changes may not be identified in the estimation of percent fat alone. The skinfold measurement is an actual measurement and not a prediction and is therefore valuable in showing body composition change. A more comprehensive evaluation can be made of the participant's progress if skinfolds are taken at several locations on the body. When these results are plotted on a norm scale, the changes that have occurred are visible and easily interpreted by the participant.

Descriptions of the location of skinfold measurements and the technique used in measuring are given next. Although only three or four sites are used in the prediction of percent body fat, other sites are necessary to use the skinfold profile.

Test Administration

Skinfolds should be taken prior to active tests because sweating and increased blood flow to the skin make measurement more difficult. Men can wear shorts for the test; women should wear shorts and a loose-fitting, sleeveless blouse or T-shirt that is also loose at the waist or the top to a two-piece swimsuit. Appropriate clothing is essential for getting accurate skinfold measurements.

Equipment

The following equipment is necessary for administering the skinfold test:

1. A skinfold caliper that conforms to specifications established by the committee of the Food and Nutrition Board of the National Research Council of the United States. The Lange and Harpenden calipers meet these specifications (see figures 6.1 and 6.2 on page 113).
2. Testing forms to record data.
3. Percent fat and target weight tables.

Different types of calipers can produce considerably different measurements. The two types used by most YMCAs are the Lange and the Harpenden. The standard pressure established for skinfold calipers is 10 g/mm² (10 grams of pressure for each square millimeter of caliper jaw surface). The Harpenden has a jaw surface of 90 mm² and the Lange, 30 mm². This means that the Harpenden has a total pressure of 900 g and the Lange, 300 g. The difference is supposedly accounted for by the distribution of pressure over the jaw surface, but the total pressure apparently does result in different measurements when calipers are compared.

Two studies (Golding 1988; Gruber and Pollock 1988) investigated these differences in calipers, and the authors found that corrections could be made to make the readings the same. When the measurement, using the Harpenden, is less than 15 mm, add one mm to each measurement; when the measurement is more than 15 mm, add 2 mm to each measurement.

When Jackson and Pollock did the research that resulted in the norms included in this book, they used Lange skinfold calipers; the tables and norms in this book were based on Lange measurements. As noted, 85% of the YMCAs reporting measurements for this book used Lange calipers.

Procedure

Taking skinfolds requires practice to ensure reliability and validity, as previously stated. Here are some suggestions on how to do it:

- Take all measurements on the person's right side.
- The easiest technique is to use two hands.
- Grasp the fold of skin firmly between the thumb and four fingers, then lift it up. Lift the fold up several times until the fold of skin and fat is picked up consistently (be certain that you have not grasped any muscle).
- Remove the right hand and replace it with the calipers, keeping the calipers close to the thumb and index finger of the left hand. A certain firmness is required to lift the skinfold accurately.
- Release the grip on the caliper completely, allowing the spring to compress the fold. Do not let go of the fold.
- Read the skinfold thickness. When the movement of the needle on the caliper dial stops, take the reading to the nearest half-millimeter. (Note: The Harpenden caliper needle makes more than one revolution; the small pointer on the dial indicates the number of revolutions.) Keeping the left hand above the skinfold allows you to read the dial easily.
- Remove the calipers, then release the fold.

The importance of measuring skinfolds accurately cannot be overemphasized. Even after extensive practice, it is possible to make errors due to slight misplacement of the caliper or misreading of the dial. The following procedure is recommended:

1. The person measuring the skinfolds should not be the one recording them. An assistant should record the values as the measurer reads the caliper measurement. It is helpful if the assistant repeats the values aloud as they are recorded.
2. It is desirable to mark each site with a marker so that the exact locations are identified. The skinfold sites can then be measured without further feeling for and trying to determine the site.
3. Skinfolds should be lifted two or three times to determine the fold to be measured before placing the calipers. Too many individuals are overly anxious to put the calipers in place before determining what really should be measured.
4. Place the calipers below the thumb and four fingers and read the dial. Repeat this movement and again lift the fold two or three times, noting the reading on the caliper dial. Unless each measurement is close (1 to 2 mm), the readings will not be consistent, and reliability will be poor.
5. If several trials result in similar measurements, record the last measurement or the measurement that occurs twice.
6. Do not lift the skinfold on the actual measurement site, as the calipers will be too far forward. The jaws of the caliper must be on the exact site. Adjust finger grip as necessary.

Locations for skinfold measurements are described in the following text and are illustrated in figures 6.4 through 6.17, which show the sites where measurements are taken.

- *Chest (pectoral)*: A diagonal fold on the pectoral line midway between the axillary fold and the nipple for men; one-third of that distance for women (figures 6.4 and 6.5)
- *Abdomen (umbilicus)*: A vertical fold approximately 1.5 in. to the right of the umbilicus (figures 6.6 and 6.7)
- *Hip (ilium or suprailium)*: A diagonal fold just above the crest of the ilium (i.e., the highest peak on the side of the pelvic girdle and on the midaxillary line) (figures 6.8 and 6.9)
- *Side (axilla, midaxilla)*: A vertical fold on the midaxillary line at nipple level (midsternum) (figures 6.10 and 6.11)
- *Arm (triceps)*: A vertical fold on the back of the upper arm midway between the shoulder and elbow joints (figures 6.12 and 6.13)
- *Back (scapula, subscapula)*: A diagonal fold on the inferior angle of the scapula (figures 6.14 and 6.15)
- *Thigh (leg)*: A vertical fold on the front of the thigh midway between the groin line and the top of the patella (kneecap) (figures 6.16 and 6.17)

Skinfold measurement results can be compared to the norm scales on the Body Composition Profile forms in appendix B. If Harpenden calipers are used, make the correction previously discussed before determining percent fat. The YMCA norms are developed for the seven sites just described. Other sites can be used, and the sites the YMCA recommends are not necessarily right and the others wrong or visa versa; they are just different. Keep in mind, however, that YMCA norms are based on the sites and the techniques we have listed here. Taking other site measurements will require getting norms for those sites.

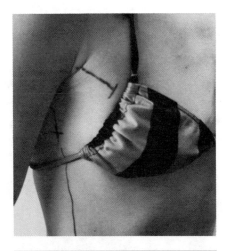

Figure 6.4 Location of pectoral skinfold.

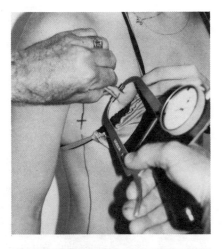

Figure 6.5 Measurement of pectoral skinfold.

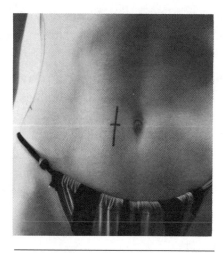

Figure 6.6 Location of abdominal skinfold.

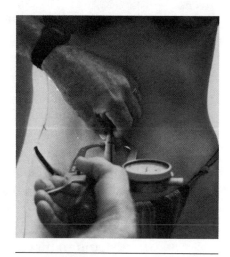

Figure 6.7 Measurement of abdominal skinfold.

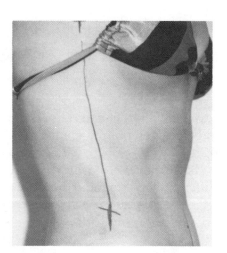

Figure 6.8 Location of hip skinfold.

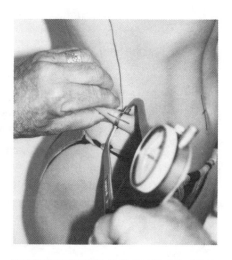

Figure 6.9 Measurement of hip skinfold.

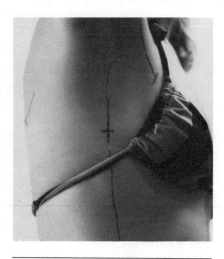

Figure 6.10 Location of axilla skinfold.

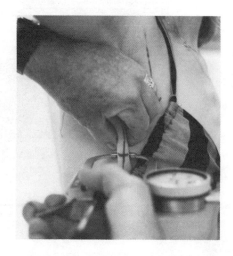

Figure 6.11 Measurement of axilla skinfold.

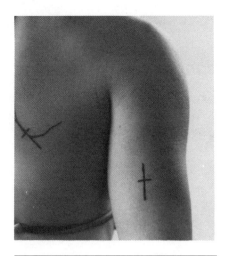

Figure 6.12 Location of triceps skinfold.

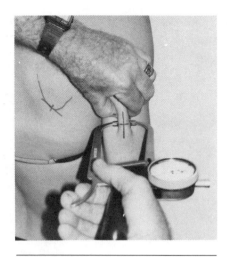

Figure 6.13 Measurement of triceps skinfold.

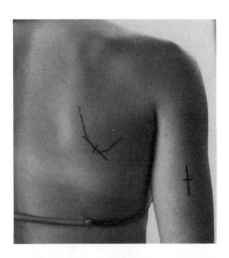

Figure 6.14 Location of scapula skinfold.

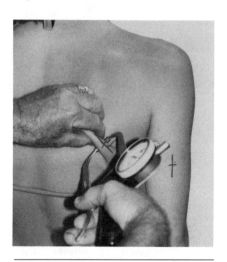

Figure 6.15 Measurement of scapula skinfold.

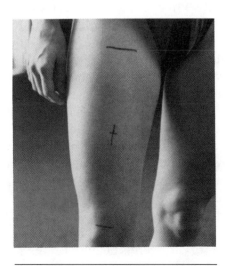

Figure 6.16 Location of thigh skinfold.

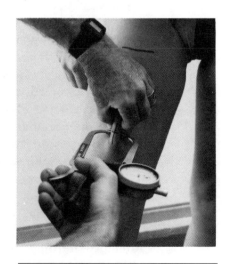

Figure 6.17 Measurement of thigh skinfold.

Using YMCA Fitness Analyst

Recording Body Composition Scores

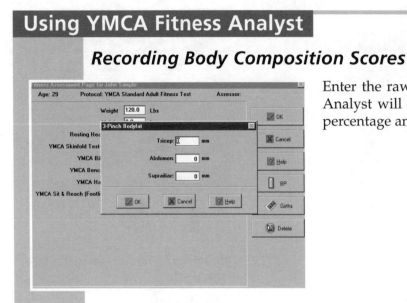

Enter the raw data and YMCA Fitness Analyst will convert them to body fat percentage and ranking.

Tests of Cardiorespiratory Endurance

Cardiorespiratory assessments are administered as field tests and through laboratory methods. The field tests are typically a distance run: Cooper's 12-Minute Run, the Mile Run, the 1.5-Mile Run, the 600-Yard Walk/Run (AAHPERD), and the Quarter-Mile Walk from the AAHPERD Older Adults Test Battery. Field tests have been widely used in Physical Ability Tests as a cardiorespiratory screening tool for groups such as firefighters, police recruits, rangers, etc. Many of these running tests have correlated well with proven laboratory tests such as maximum oxygen uptake. The advantage of field tests is that little or no testing equipment is needed (shoes, a measured course, and a stopwatch). Large numbers of individuals can be tested at one time. The New York City Fire Department may get as many as 15,000 applicants for a firefighter position opening, and all of these have to take the fire department's Physical Abilities Test (PAT). It is inconceivable to attempt to test this number of people individually. The "run" can be used to test as many as 25 or 50 individuals at one time. Usually the test has a minimum time for the run, and after that time has expired, the balance of the runners fail the test. Another advantage of the field test is that no skilled or trained technicians are needed to administer it.

When a certain level of fitness is required for a job, such as firefighting, litigation problems related to how the cut-off time was established to determine whether the person can or cannot do the tasks required by the job may occur. Most litigation that has occurred is due to an inability to justify why a particular cut-off time was chosen. Is it really fair that one individual with a time of 8 minutes is identified as able to perform the job, whereas another with a time of 8:01 is considered unable?

The disadvantage of field tests is that temperature, wind, and humidity can seldom be controlled, and these factors can weigh heavily on the results of the run. In addition, group running often establishes a competitive atmosphere that can influence some to overexert themselves dangerously.

The laboratory assessment of cardiorespiratory fitness has been done for years. Most of the laboratory tests use either heart rate (exercise HR or recovery HR), oxygen uptake, or predictions of maximum oxygen uptake.

The early cardiorespiratory tests were step tests. These tests only required a sturdy bench of a required height, a stethoscope, a stopwatch, a metronome, and a timer. Even pulse-rate counting sometimes replaced the stethoscope. The height of the bench and the metronome to control the speed of stepping determined the amount of work that was being performed. Because step tests were done indoors, environmental conditions such as temperature and wind could be controlled. The heart rate measured was the recovery heart rate, which was taken after the person stopped stepping. The score was based on the principle that the quicker the heart rate returned to its pre-exercise level, the fitter the individual.

The disadvantage of the step test is that the weight of subjects differs, so that a heavy individual is doing much more work than a lighter individual. This limitation is not as important when comparing pre- and posttraining results for the same individual, but it is limiting when using norm tables based on a large population. The height of the individual also imposes a limitation. A subject who is 80-inches tall is mechanically at an advantage over another subject whose height is 60 inches. Because the norm tables used with step tests involved large numbers of individuals, the variation in height and weight was ignored.

Although not used as much today there were several well-used and well-researched step tests: the Harvard Step Test (a 5-minute step test), the Tuttle Step Tests, the Progressive Pulse Ratio Test, the Ohio State Step Test, and several others. Later in this chapter we discuss the YMCA's 3-Minute Step Test (Kasch step test) in more detail.

Treadmills have been used in laboratories since the early Harvard Fatigue Laboratory days. The treadmill allows an individual to walk or run at a prescribed speed and grade and can be easily adjusted for both. The subject can perform at the same workload, under the same conditions, whenever desired. Because the subject remains in the same place, various measurements can be taken easily while the subject is running. ECGs, blood pressure, blood samples, and oxygen uptake can all be successfully measured even when the subject is performing maximally. When cardiologists began using graded exercise testing (GXT) to diagnose heart disease, the treadmill was chosen as the choice ergometer. In Europe, however, the cycle ergometer was more popular. Europeans used the bicycle more in everyday life whereas the Americans did not. GXTs are easily administered by simply increasing speed or grade, or both, and these increases can be done in small increments. Changes in the patient's adaptation to exercise or changes in the ECG can be detected as soon as they happen, and exercise can be stopped or reduced immediately.

Most step tests, because of the height of the bench and the speed of stepping, did not allow the subject to increase or decrease the workload easily. The Master's Step Test, which before treadmills was considered to be the gold standard in exercise testing, had the subject exercise and then after the subject completed the stepping the ECG was administered. The Master's Step Test, however, had no provisions for monitoring if and when a subject began to have difficulty during the stepping. Some step tests did try to vary the workload by varying the speed of stepping or changing the height of the bench. Cureton's Progressive Pulse Ratio Test, which was used by the YMCA for years, used a stepping rate that increased from 12 steps per minute to 18, to 24, to 30, and to 36. The Ohio State

Step Test had a bench made like a staircase with three stepping heights, and the subject moved from one height bench to the next higher bench and so on.

Despite the drawbacks of step testing, the treadmill was not the ideal solution for cardiorespiratory testing. The treadmill is usually large, heavy, expensive, and requires a fairly large space. Treadmills are also seldom portable. In addition, when the first tests were developed, treadmills were not as prevalent in YMCAs as they are today.

When the cycle ergometer was finally introduced, a new dimension to cardiorespiratory assessment began. The cycle ergometer is less expensive than the treadmill, it requires less space, and it is easily transported. In addition, subjects do not usually require a practice session. Like the treadmill, workloads can be increased in small increments; a speedometer, or a metronome, keeps the speed of pedaling constant; and because the upper body is stationary, measurements such as blood pressure and the extracting of blood are easier to take than on the treadmill. The cycle ergometer has an additional benefit; namely, body weight is not a factor because the activity is nonweightbearing. In both stepping and treadmill work, body weight plays an important role in the amount of work performed. This advantage is important when assessing an obese individual or an older adult.

In the YMCA Fitness Assessment protocol, the cycle ergometer was selected to evaluate the participant's cardiorespiratory fitness. The test is used with the understanding that the participant has no medical contraindications to participate in fitness testing and a subsequent exercise program.

The cycle test, which predicts maximum working capacity by measuring the response to submaximal work, can also be used as a means of predicting maximum oxygen consumption. The latter is an additional measurement that can be determined from the results of the test without any further testing.

A step test is also available for use by YMCA fitness specialists in group testing. It is an excellent substitute for the cycle ergometer test when the amount of equipment and number of staff are insufficient for administering individual tests. The step test is discussed later.

It is desirable for participants in their first year of fitness training to repeat testing once after about 10 to 12 weeks and then again at the end of 6 to 12 months. Repeat testing shows participants their personal responses to training and may possibly act as a motivator for continued participation. After the first year of participation in a fitness program, most individuals need not be tested more than once a year.

The measurements resulting from the cycle test reflect the cardiorespiratory response of the individual to increasing amounts of work and should be used to show changes in endurance during the exercise training program. If an individual scores in either the fair or poor categories of the cycle test (see Physical Fitness Evaluation Profile for rating scales), he or she should start out more slowly in an exercise program than those scoring average or above. These individuals may not have the cardiorespiratory capacity to perform moderate to strenuous work and may start out with a walking program for several weeks before beginning more intense exercise. In any case, signs of overexertion should be monitored during the first few weeks of one's program. Individuals who score in the average, good, or excellent categories should be able to handle a properly designed exercise program commensurate with their fitness rating.

The two tests presently used in the YMCA Fitness Assessment protocol are the YMCA Physical Working Capacity Maximum Test and the 3-Minute Step Test.

YMCA Maximum Physical Working Capacity Test (PWCmax)

When developing this fitness assessment battery for the YMCA, the originators chose to use a cycle ergometer rather than a treadmill for the cardiorespiratory endurance test. They recognized that the cycle offered several advantages over a treadmill:

- Less expensive
- Requires little space
- Easily transported
- Easier to take heart rate
- External workloads are expressed scientifically (kgm)

Until the YMCA started using the PWCmax test, the most commonly used tests on the cycle were the PWC 170 as developed by Sjostrand (1947) and the estimation of maximum oxygen uptake by Åstrand and Rhyming (1954). Both tests are based on the fact that heart rate and oxygen uptake are linear functions of the rate of work. In the Åstrand and Rhyming test the purpose was to estimate the individual's maximal oxygen uptake ($\dot{V}O_2$max) from the submaximal cycle test. Maximum oxygen uptake is highly related to the individual's capacity for heavy prolonged work.

A linear relationship exists between heart rate (HR) and work (W); however, this linearity exists only at certain heart rates. At low heart rates, many external stimuli can affect the heart rate (e.g., talking, laughter, nervousness). However, once the muscles demand more blood and the blood is shunted to the working muscles, the heart starts pumping harder and external stimuli no longer influence the heart rate causing linearity; this situation occurs at about 110 beats/min. The relationship between heart rate and work increases in a linear fashion until it plateaus, signaling the maximum heart rate. A 70-year-old person will plateau (reach max HR) at about 150, and because most cycle test subjects will be less than 70 years old, it is assumed that the vast majority of participants will be linear between 110 and 150 beats/min (see figure 6.18).

The basis of the PWCmax test is to establish, for the individual being tested, the line between heart rate and work. To establish a line, a minimum of two points is needed; therefore the HRs at two workloads are used. The only precaution is that these two points must be in the linear portion of the relationship. The workloads cannot be too high or too low or they may fall into the nonlinear portion of the relationship.

As stated, linearity begins at approximately 110 beats/min. The plateau after reaching maximum heart rate is a function of age; however, at a heart rate of 150 beats/min, almost everyone tested will still be linear. Therefore, linearity is said to be between 110 and 150 beats/min.

To eliminate the need to guess the workload required to start the test, a guide to setting workloads is presented in figure 6.19. By following the guidelines

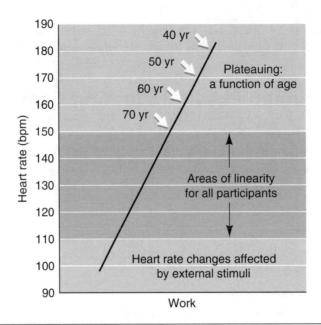

Figure 6.18 Linear relationship between heart rate and work.

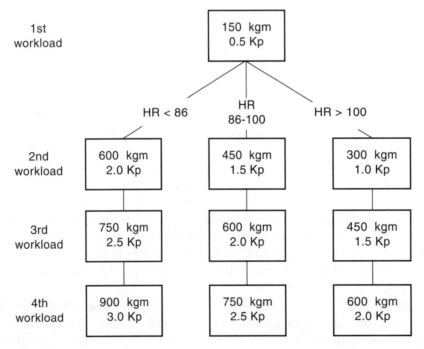

Directions:

1. Set the first workload at 150 kgm/min (0.5 Kp).

2. If the HR in the third min is
   - less than 86, set the second load at 600 kgm (2.0 Kp);
   - 86 to 100, set the second load at 450 kgm (1.5 Kp);
   - greater than 100, set the second load at 300 kgm (1.0 Kp).

3. Set the third and fourth (if required) loads according to the loads in the columns below the second loads.

Figure 6.19 Guide to setting workloads on a cycle ergometer.

suggested in the figure, a tester should be able to eliminate the possibility of presenting the participant with too difficult a workload. The workload chart should be used conservatively, as it is better to give too small rather than too large a workload.

The first workload is given to determine the heart-rate response elicited for a small workload. Usually the first workload will not be plotted because the heart rate will be under 110 beats/min; however, should the heart rate rise above 110 beats/min, the first workload should be plotted. Then only one more workload will be necessary to plot the line between two points. If the heart rate is not 110 beats/min or greater, then two more workloads will be necessary to plot two points.

Many laboratories doing research use three plot points. Because these three points are seldom plotted on an exact line, a line of best fit must be computed. No significant difference has been found between using two points or three or more points.

As part of understanding the bicycle test, the concepts of steady-state heart rate, maximum heart rate, and maximum oxygen uptake should be understood. Following is a quick review.

Steady-State Heart Rate. The moment a participant starts to work, the heart rate immediately increases. At the end of a minute of work, the heart rate is still increasing. It takes about three minutes of work before the heart rate stabilizes. This state of plateau is called the steady-state heart rate. (See discussion on page 60.)

Although steady-state heart rate usually occurs within three minutes, it may take longer. If the difference between the second-minute heart rate and the third-minute heart rate is more than five beats/min, the heart rate is still significantly increasing, and a fourth minute should be added. If the difference is five or less beats/min, the heart rate has stabilized.

When the workload is increased, the same sequence occurs to establish a steady-state heart rate at the new, increased workload. As the test needs to be kept as short as possible, accuracy can be maintained by having the participant pedal for 3 minutes at each workload with no rests between workloads. Figures 6.20 and 6.21 illustrate the heart rate changes in response to a progressive bicycle ergometer test. The steady-state heart rate (SSHR) in figure 6.20 is used to plot the heart rate in figure 6.21, which determines the physical working capacity (PWC) value. The graph is drawn on the assumption that the heart rate at the first workload was less than 110 beats/min and therefore is outside the linear portion of the curve. Only the second and third workloads were plotted.

Maximum Heart Rate. As an individual works harder, the heart rate increases in a linear fashion—the higher the workload, the higher the heart rate. At some point, even though the amount of work increases, the heart rate does not increase. At this point the heart has reached its fastest rate or maximum heart rate. Everyone has a point at which the heart rate will go no higher, although this point differs among individuals for various reasons. The main reason is age. As one ages, the ability to drive the heart to high rates decreases. This decrease in maximum heart rate is partly due to a decrease in physical fitness, and in the general population this decrease is very evident. In fit individuals who continue aerobic activity into later life, however, the decrease is not so rapid.

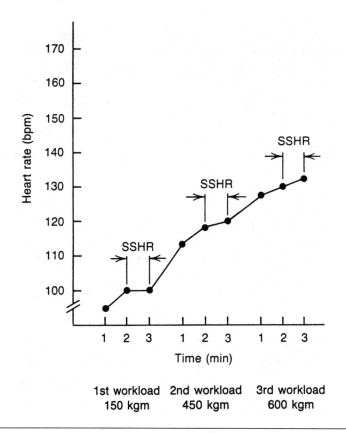

Figure 6.20 Example of heart rate changes during the cycle ergometer test.

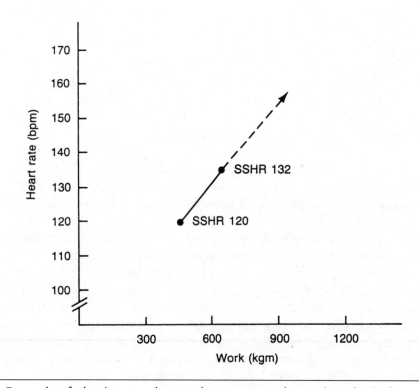

Figure 6.21 Example of plotting steady-state heart rate to determine physical working capacity.

It has been shown that maximum heart rate decreases with age in a linear fashion as was depicted in figure 4.13 on page 62. The formula of 220 minus age predicts an individual's maximum heart rate. A 40-year-old male would have a predicted maximum heart rate of 180. This prediction is only representative of the average for a population of 40-year-old males and does not take into account individual variations.

Maximum Oxygen Uptake ($\dot{V}O_2$max). The maximum oxygen uptake is an excellent test of cardiorespiratory efficiency and is often mentioned in both scientific and popular literature. The measurement of maximum oxygen uptake is a laboratory technique that involves both the collection and the analysis of expired air during exercise; however, because it is known that both heart rate and oxygen uptake have a linear relationship to workload, it is possible to predict the maximum oxygen uptake. As the workload increases, the heart rate and the oxygen uptake increase. This relationship allows the prediction of a maximum oxygen uptake from the maximum heart rate. (See discussion of oxygen uptake on page 73.)

The cycle ergometer test shows the relationship of heart rate to work and thereby can predict the workload that an individual would be capable of handling at maximum heart rate. It can also be used to predict an individual's maximum oxygen uptake.

The amount of oxygen needed for any task is a function of size (i.e., weight), so oxygen uptakes among individuals, including males and females, can be compared only if their weights are equalized. Weight equalization is accomplished by dividing oxygen uptake by body weight. *Note*: For ease of calculation, convert oxygen uptake from liters per minute (L · min⁻¹) to milliliters per minute (ml · min⁻¹) by multiplying by 1000 or by moving the decimal point three places to the right. Divide by body weight in kilograms (divide 1 lb by 2.2 to get kg) to obtain results in milliliters per kilogram (milliliters divided by kilograms = ml/kg). Because oxygen uptake is always given per minute, this expression becomes ml/kg/min, or ml · kg⁻¹ · min⁻¹ (see the $\dot{V}O_2$ conversion chart in table 6.10).

Test Administration

On the day of testing the participant should abstain from any physical exertion and from smoking or eating for two hours prior to the test. The cycle test is administered in the same manner for both men and women.

Metronomes

A few comments about the use of a metronome may be appropriate. A metronome is required to administer the cycle ergometer test and is also required for the bench press and step tests. There are two kinds of metronomes: mechanical and electrical. Mechanical metronomes typically have a wand that moves from side to side. The cadence is changed by moving a weight up or down the wand. Mechanical metronomes must be manually wound to operate. Electrical metronomes have both an auditory and a visual signal and do not need to be wound.

Both types of metronomes need to be calibrated. Calibrate by timing the number of beats with a stopwatch. If a metronome is set for 100 beats/min, it may be tested by counting the number of beats in 30 seconds and multiplying by 2. If fewer than 50 beats occur in 30 seconds, move the weight down the wand; if more than 50 beats occur, move the weight up the wand. Time the beats again, making adjustments until the cadence matches the time.

Table 6.10 Maximum Oxygen Uptake Conversion Chart (L/kg/min to mL/kg/min)

Body weight		Maximum oxygen uptake (L/kg/min)																																													
lb	kg	1.5	1.6	1.7	1.8	1.9	2.0	2.1	2.2	2.3	2.4	2.5	2.6	2.7	2.8	2.9	3.0	3.1	3.2	3.3	3.4	3.5	3.6	3.7	3.8	3.9	4.0	4.1	4.2	4.3	4.4	4.5	4.6	4.7	4.8	4.9	5.0	5.1	5.2	5.3	5.4	5.5	5.6	5.7	5.8	5.9	6.0
110	50	30	32	34	36	38	40	42	44	46	48	50	52	54	56	58	60	62	64	66	68	70	72	74	76	78	80	82	84	86	88	90	92	94	96	98	100	102	104	106	108	110	112	114	116	118	120
112	51	29	31	33	35	37	39	41	43	45	47	49	51	53	55	57	59	61	63	65	67	69	71	73	75	76	78	80	82	84	86	88	90	92	94	93	98	100	102	104	106	108	110	112	114	116	118
115	52	29	31	33	35	37	38	40	42	44	46	48	50	52	54	56	58	60	62	63	65	67	69	71	73	75	77	79	81	83	85	87	88	90	92	94	96	98	100	102	104	106	108	110	112	113	115
117	53	28	30	32	34	36	38	40	42	43	45	47	49	51	53	55	57	58	60	62	64	66	68	70	72	74	75	77	79	81	83	85	87	89	91	92	94	96	98	100	102	104	106	108	109	111	113
119	54	28	30	31	33	35	37	39	41	43	44	46	48	50	52	54	56	57	59	61	63	65	67	69	70	72	74	76	78	80	81	83	85	87	89	91	96	94	96	98	100	102	104	106	107	109	111
121	55	27	29	31	33	35	36	38	40	42	44	45	47	49	51	53	55	56	58	60	62	64	65	67	69	71	73	75	76	78	80	82	84	85	87	89	91	93	95	96	98	100	102	104	105	107	109
123	56	27	29	30	32	34	36	38	39	41	43	45	46	48	50	52	54	55	57	59	61	63	64	66	68	70	71	73	75	77	79	80	82	84	86	88	89	91	93	95	96	98	100	102	104	105	107
126	57	26	28	30	32	33	35	37	39	41	42	44	46	47	49	51	53	54	56	58	60	61	63	65	67	68	70	72	74	75	77	79	81	82	84	86	88	89	91	93	95	96	98	100	102	104	105
128	58	26	28	29	31	33	34	36	38	40	41	43	45	47	48	50	52	53	55	57	59	60	62	64	65	67	69	71	72	74	76	78	79	81	83	84	85	88	90	91	93	95	97	98	100	102	103
130	59	25	27	29	31	32	34	36	37	39	41	42	44	46	47	49	51	53	54	56	58	59	61	63	64	65	68	69	71	73	75	76	78	80	81	83	85	86	88	90	92	93	95	97	98	100	102
132	60	25	27	28	30	32	33	35	37	38	40	42	43	45	47	48	50	52	53	55	57	58	60	62	63	65	67	68	70	72	73	75	77	78	80	82	83	85	87	88	90	92	93	95	97	98	100
134	61	25	26	28	30	31	33	34	36	38	39	41	43	44	46	48	49	51	52	54	56	57	59	61	62	64	66	67	69	70	72	74	75	77	79	80	82	84	85	87	89	90	92	96	95	97	98
137	62	24	26	27	29	31	32	34	35	37	39	40	42	44	45	47	48	50	52	53	55	56	58	60	61	63	65	66	68	69	71	73	74	76	77	79	81	82	84	85	87	89	90	92	94	95	97
139	63	24	25	27	29	30	32	33	35	37	38	40	41	43	44	46	48	49	51	52	54	56	57	59	60	62	63	65	67	68	70	71	73	75	76	78	79	81	83	84	86	87	89	90	92	94	95
141	64	23	25	27	28	30	31	33	34	36	38	39	41	42	44	45	47	48	50	52	53	55	56	58	59	61	63	64	66	67	69	70	72	73	75	77	78	80	81	83	84	86	88	89	91	92	94
143	65	23	25	26	28	29	31	32	34	35	37	38	40	42	43	45	46	48	49	51	52	54	55	57	58	60	62	63	65	66	68	69	71	72	74	75	77	78	80	82	83	85	86	88	89	91	92
146	66	23	24	26	27	29	30	32	33	35	36	38	39	41	42	44	45	47	48	50	52	53	55	56	58	59	61	62	64	65	67	68	70	71	73	74	76	77	79	80	82	83	85	86	88	89	91
148	67	22	24	25	27	28	30	31	33	34	36	37	39	40	42	43	45	46	48	49	51	52	54	55	57	58	60	61	63	64	66	67	69	70	72	73	75	76	78	79	81	82	84	82	87	88	90
150	68	22	24	25	26	28	29	31	32	34	35	37	38	40	41	43	44	46	47	49	50	51	53	54	56	57	59	60	62	63	65	66	68	69	71	72	74	75	76	78	79	81	82	84	85	87	88
152	69	22	23	25	26	28	29	30	32	33	35	36	38	39	41	42	43	45	46	48	49	51	52	54	55	57	58	59	61	62	64	65	67	68	70	71	72	74	75	77	78	80	81	86	84	86	87
154	70	21	23	24	26	27	29	30	31	33	34	36	37	39	40	41	43	44	46	47	49	50	51	53	54	56	57	59	60	61	63	64	66	67	69	70	71	73	74	76	77	79	80	81	83	84	86
157	71	21	23	24	25	27	28	30	31	32	34	35	37	38	39	41	42	44	45	46	48	49	51	52	54	55	56	58	59	61	62	63	65	66	68	69	70	72	73	75	76	77	79	80	82	83	85
159	72	21	22	24	25	26	28	29	31	32	33	35	36	38	39	40	42	43	44	46	47	49	50	51	53	54	56	57	58	60	61	63	64	65	67	68	69	71	72	74	75	76	78	79	81	82	83
161	73	21	22	23	25	26	27	29	30	32	33	34	36	37	38	40	41	42	44	45	47	48	49	51	52	53	55	56	58	59	60	62	63	64	66	67	68	70	71	73	74	75	77	78	79	81	82
163	74	20	22	23	24	26	27	28	30	31	32	34	35	36	38	39	41	42	43	45	46	47	49	50	54	53	54	55	57	58	59	61	62	64	65	65	68	69	70	72	73	74	76	77	78	80	81
165	75	20	21	23	24	25	27	28	29	31	32	33	35	36	37	39	40	41	43	44	45	47	48	49	51	52	53	55	56	57	59	60	61	63	64	65	67	68	69	71	72	73	75	76	77	79	80
168	76	20	21	22	24	25	26	28	29	30	32	33	34	36	37	38	39	41	42	43	45	46	47	49	50	51	53	54	55	57	58	59	61	62	63	64	66	67	68	70	71	72	74	75	76	78	79
170	77	19	21	22	23	25	26	27	29	30	31	32	34	35	36	38	39	40	42	43	44	45	47	48	49	51	52	53	55	56	57	58	60	61	62	64	65	66	68	69	70	71	73	74	75	77	78
172	78	19	21	22	23	24	26	27	28	29	31	32	33	35	36	37	38	40	41	42	44	45	46	47	49	50	51	53	54	55	56	58	59	60	62	63	64	68	67	68	69	71	72	73	74	76	77
174	79	19	20	22	23	24	25	27	28	29	30	32	33	34	35	37	38	39	41	42	43	44	46	47	48	49	51	52	53	54	56	57	58	59	61	62	63	65	66	67	68	70	71	72	73	75	76
176	80	19	20	21	23	24	25	26	28	29	30	31	33	34	35	36	38	39	40	41	43	44	45	46	48	49	50	51	53	54	55	56	58	59	60	61	63	64	65	66	68	69	70	71	72	74	75
179	81	19	20	21	22	23	25	26	27	28	30	31	32	33	35	36	37	38	40	41	42	46	44	46	47	48	49	51	52	53	54	56	57	58	59	60	62	63	64	65	67	68	69	71	72	73	74
181	82	18	20	21	22	23	24	26	27	28	29	30	32	33	34	35	37	38	39	40	41	43	44	45	46	48	49	50	51	52	54	55	56	57	59	60	61	62	63	65	66	67	68	70	71	72	73
183	83	18	19	20	22	23	24	25	27	28	29	30	31	33	34	35	36	37	39	40	41	42	43	45	46	47	48	49	51	52	53	54	55	57	58	59	60	61	63	64	65	66	67	69	70	71	72
185	84	18	19	20	21	23	24	25	26	27	29	30	31	32	33	35	36	37	38	39	40	42	43	44	45	46	48	49	50	51	52	54	55	56	57	58	60	61	62	63	64	65	67	68	69	70	71
187	85	18	19	20	21	22	24	25	26	27	28	29	31	32	33	34	35	36	38	39	40	41	42	44	45	46	47	48	49	51	52	53	54	55	56	58	59	60	61	62	64	65	66	67	68	69	71
190	86	17	19	20	21	22	23	24	26	27	28	29	30	31	33	34	35	36	37	38	40	41	42	43	44	45	47	48	49	50	51	52	53	55	56	57	58	59	60	62	63	64	65	66	67	69	70
192	87	17	18	20	21	22	23	24	25	26	28	29	30	31	32	33	34	36	37	38	39	40	41	43	44	45	46	47	48	49	51	52	53	54	55	56	57	59	60	61	62	63	64	66	67	68	69
194	88	17	18	19	20	22	23	24	25	26	27	28	30	31	32	33	34	35	36	38	39	40	41	42	43	44	45	47	48	49	50	51	52	53	55	56	57	58	59	60	61	63	64	65	65	67	68
196	89	17	18	19	20	21	22	24	25	26	27	28	29	30	31	33	34	35	36	37	38	39	40	42	43	44	45	46	47	48	49	51	52	53	54	55	56	57	58	60	61	62	63	64	65	66	67
198	90	17	18	19	20	21	22	23	24	26	27	28	29	30	31	32	33	34	36	37	38	39	40	41	42	43	44	46	47	48	49	50	51	52	53	54	56	57	58	59	60	61	62	63	64	66	67
201	91	16	18	19	20	21	22	23	24	25	26	27	29	30	31	32	33	34	35	36	37	38	40	41	42	43	44	45	46	47	48	49	51	52	53	54	55	56	57	58	59	60	62	63	64	65	66
203	92	16	17	18	20	21	22	23	24	25	26	27	28	29	30	32	33	34	35	36	37	38	39	40	41	42	43	45	46	47	48	49	50	51	52	53	54	55	57	58	59	60	61	62	63	64	65
205	93	16	17	18	19	20	22	23	24	25	26	27	28	29	30	31	32	33	34	35	37	38	39	40	41	42	43	44	45	46	47	48	49	51	52	53	54	55	56	57	58	59	60	61	62	63	65
207	94	16	17	18	19	20	21	22	23	24	26	27	28	29	30	31	32	33	34	35	36	37	38	39	40	41	43	44	45	46	47	48	49	50	51	52	53	54	55	56	57	59	60	61	62	63	64
209	95	16	17	18	19	20	21	22	23	24	25	26	27	28	29	31	32	33	34	35	36	37	38	39	40	41	42	43	44	45	46	47	48	49	51	52	53	54	55	56	57	58	59	60	61	62	63
212	96	16	17	18	19	20	21	22	23	24	25	26	27	28	29	30	31	32	33	34	35	36	38	39	40	41	42	43	44	45	46	47	48	49	50	51	52	53	54	55	56	57	58	59	60	61	63
214	97	15	16	18	19	20	21	22	23	24	25	26	27	28	29	30	31	32	33	34	35	36	37	38	39	40	41	42	43	44	45	46	47	48	49	51	52	53	54	55	56	57	58	59	60	61	62
216	98	15	16	17	18	19	20	21	22	23	24	26	27	28	29	30	31	32	33	34	35	36	37	38	39	40	41	42	43	44	45	46	47	48	49	50	51	52	53	54	55	56	57	58	59	60	61
218	99	15	16	17	18	19	20	21	22	23	24	25	26	27	28	29	30	31	32	33	34	35	36	37	38	39	40	41	42	43	44	45	46	47	48	49	51	52	53	54	55	56	57	58	59	60	61
220	100	15	16	17	18	19	20	21	22	23	24	25	26	27	28	29	30	31	32	33	34	35	36	37	38	39	40	41	42	43	44	45	46	47	48	49	50	51	52	53	54	55	56	57	58	59	60

Reprinted by permission from *Work Tests with the Bicycle Ergometer* (p. 14) P.-O. Åstrand, n.d., Varberg, Sweden: Monark. Copyright by Monark AB.

Metronomes usually have no volume control and are often too quiet for testing. One answer to this problem is to make an audiotape recording of the metronome and use the recording during testing sessions. Recording allows for volume control and makes a very efficient metronome. Three 60-minute tapes are recommended: one at 60 beats/min (bench press test), one at 96 beats/min (step test), and one at 100 beats/min (cycle test). These three tapes supply all the metronome needs for the test battery and eliminate any need for future calibration.

Workload Guide

The workload guide was developed to help in the administration of the cycle ergometer test. Set the initial workload at 150 kilogram-meters per minute (kgm/min) (see figure 6.19 for workload guidelines). On the Monark ergometer, one complete turn of the pedals on the bicycle moves the wheel 6 m. At a pedaling rate of 50 rpm (revolutions per minute), the total distance covered in one minute is 300 m. If the scale is set so that 1 kg of force is acting on the wheel, then 300m/min · 1 kg = 300 kgm/min. Table 6.11 gives the workload in kgm/min for each scale setting on the Monark cycle ergometer.

Table 6.11 Scale Setting and Workload on Cycle Ergometer

Scale setting	Workload (kgm/min)	Scale setting	Workload (kgm/min)
0.5 Kp	150	4.0 Kp	1200
1.0 Kp	300	4.5 Kp	1350
1.5 Kp	450	5.0 Kp	1500
2.0 Kp	600	5.5 Kp	1650
2.5 Kp	750	6.0 Kp	1800
3.0 Kp	900	6.5 Kp	1950
3.5 Kp	1050	7.0 Kp	2100

Equipment

The following equipment is necessary for the cycle ergometer test:

1. An accurate, easily calibrated, constant torque cycle ergometer with a range of 0 to 2100 kgm/min (see figure 6.22). A kilogram-meter is a unit of work that is equal to the energy required to lift 1 kg (2.2 lb) vertically a distance of 1 m (3.3 ft). Each major graduation is 300 kgm, with intermediate marks at 150 kgm. Because the Monark cycle ergometer is the one most commonly used in YMCAs, it is used in the following examples; other brands meeting these criteria may be used as well.

2. A metronome set at 100 beats/min.

3. A timer to clock riding duration.

4. A stopwatch to time heart rate.

5. A stethoscope to count heart rate.

6. Testing forms to record data.

Note: Resting HR and recovery HRs are not used in the cycle ergometer test.

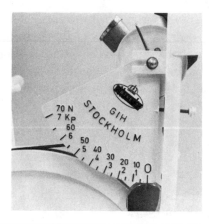

Figure 6.22 Workload scale on cycle ergometer.

Procedure

Check the calibration of the cycle. On the Monark be sure the red line on the pendulum weight reads zero on the workload scale before starting. Pedaling with no resistance, set the line at zero. Moving an adjusting wing nut easily corrects this if it is not in line (see figure 6.23 for information on calibrating the cycle). If another brand of cycle ergometer is used, follow the manufacturer's instructions for calibration. All cycles exhibit a slight difference in resistance; be sure that any retesting is done on the same bicycle.

Briefly explain the concept and the protocol of the test to the participant and fill out the test forms.

Adjust the seat height on the ergometer. When the pedal is at its lowest point the knee should be straight, with the ball of the foot on the pedal and the leg stretched. Note the seat position on the score sheet so that it may be used in retesting.

Set the metronome at either 50 or 100 beats/min and allow the participant to pedal freewheel (no load) for a minute to get the pace. At 50 revolutions per minute (rpm) the right foot makes 50 complete revolutions in one minute. The metronome set at 100 beats/min means that at each "click" a foot (left or right) should be on the downstroke. This is still 50 rpm.

Allow the participant to work at the first workload for three minutes. Count the heart rate at the second and third minutes (see figure 6.24). The difference in heart rates between the second and third minutes should not vary by more that five beats; if it does, have the participant extend the ride for an extra minute or until a stable value is obtained. With the stopwatch, time 30 heartbeats. Start the stopwatch on a beat, counting it as "zero," and stop the watch at 30 beats (see page 59 on HR counting). See the heart rate conversion chart (table 6.12) to find the HR in beats per minute. Check the steady-state heart rate against figure 6.19 as a guide to setting the workloads. Remember that the purpose of this guide is to set the task in small increments so that the workload does not cause the heart rate to increase too rapidly or to reach too high a level. Conservatism is the rule. An extra workload will not change the results of the test. Remember the test should be a submaximal test. Record the heart rate carefully.

Change the workload. There is no need to hurry to change it, as the participant may ride four or five minutes at each workload. Take time to record the heart

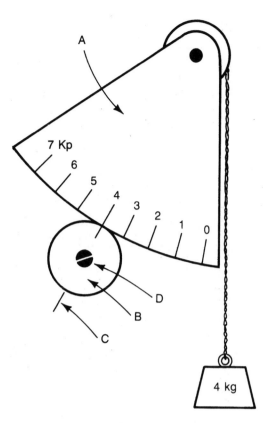

The calibration of the bike is done precisely at the factory and, unless the adjusting screw (C) has been tampered with, seldom is there a need for recalibration. However, if you suspect incorrect calibration it can be checked as follows.

Set the mark on the pendulum weight (B) at 0. Attach a weight known to be very accurate as shown above. A 1-kg weight should correspond to a reading of 1 on the scale (A); a 2-kg weight should correspond to a reading of 2 on the scale (A); and so on. The example above shows 4 kg corresponding to 4 on the scale.

If the numbers do not agree it can be corrected by changing the adjusting screw (C). This screw moves the center of gravity of the pendulum (this screw is locked with the screw D).

Figure 6.23 Cycle ergometer calibration.
Reprinted by permission from *Work Tests with the Bicycle Ergometer* (p. 14) P.-O. Åstrand, n.d., Varberg, Sweden: Monark. Copyright by Monark AB.

rate properly after each workload before putting in the next workload. Reset the clock and record the new workload on the score sheet. As each participant's second and third workloads will differ, enter these on the score sheet as soon as they are determined, to avoid errors later.

Regularly check the workload setting during each workload period. As the friction belt gets hot, it may slip, giving less resistance. Returning it to the desired workload will ensure that the participant is doing the workload that is required.

Because the steady-state heart rate is being elicited at each workload, exactly when the heart rate is taken is not critical. For consistency the heart rate should be taken as the full two- and three-minute marks are reached. This means that the participant actually rides a little longer than three minutes.

After the second workload is completed, record the heart rate at the end of the second and third minutes. Again, these should not differ by more than five beats. Unless the first workload produced a heart rate of 110 beats/min or more,

Table 6.12   Heart Rate Conversion Chart (30 beats to bpm)

Sec	bpm	Sec	bpm	Sec	bpm
22.0	82	17.3	104	12.6	143
21.9	82	17.2	105	12.5	144
21.8	83	17.1	105	12.4	145
21.7	83	17.0	106	12.3	146
21.6	83	16.9	107	12.2	148
21.5	84	16.8	107	12.1	149
21.4	84	16.7	108	12.0	150
21.3	85	16.6	108	11.9	151
21.2	85	16.5	109	11.8	153
21.1	85	16.4	110	11.7	154
21.0	86	16.3	110	11.6	155
20.9	86	16.2	111	11.5	157
20.8	87	16.1	112	11.4	158
20.7	87	16.0	113	11.3	159
20.6	87	15.9	113	11.2	161
20.5	88	15.8	114	11.1	162
20.4	88	15.7	115	11.0	164
20.3	89	15.6	115	10.9	165
20.2	89	15.5	116	10.8	167
20.1	90	15.4	117	10.7	168
20.0	90	15.3	118	10.6	170
19.9	90	15.2	118	10.5	171
19.8	91	15.1	119	10.4	173
19.7	91	15.0	120	10.3	175
19.6	92	14.9	121	10.2	176
19.5	92	14.8	122	10.1	178
19.4	93	14.7	122	10.0	180
19.3	93	14.6	123	9.9	182
19.2	94	14.5	124	9.8	184
19.1	94	14.4	125	9.7	186
19.0	95	14.3	126	9.6	188
18.9	95	14.2	127	9.5	189
18.8	96	14.1	128	9.4	191
18.7	96	14.0	129	9.3	194
18.6	97	13.9	129	9.2	196
18.5	97	13.8	130	9.1	198
18.4	98	13.7	131	9.0	200
18.3	98	13.6	132	8.9	202
18.2	99	13.5	133	8.8	205
18.1	99	13.4	134	8.7	207
18.0	100	13.3	135	8.6	209
17.9	101	13.2	136	8.5	212
17.8	101	13.1	137	8.4	214
17.7	102	13.0	138	8.3	217
17.6	102	12.9	140	8.2	220
17.5	103	12.8	141	8.1	222
17.4	103	12.7	142	8.0	225

Reprinted by permission from *Work Tests With the Bicycle Ergometer* (p.14) P.-O. Åstrand, n.d., Varberg, Sweden: Monark. Copyright by Monark AB.

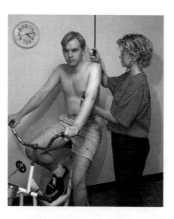

Figure 6.24   Taking heart rate on cycle ergometer.

determine the third workload and proceed. If the first workload did produce 110 beats/min, a third workload is not needed.

Throughout the test observe the participant closely for any exertional intolerance or other signs of undue fatigue or unusual response. Instruct the participant to indicate how he or she feels from time to time. However, do not engage the participant in conversation during the testing.

Record the heart rate at the end of the second and third minutes of the third workload. The test is now complete. Have the participant cool down by riding at no resistance.

Scoring

Once the test is complete, the final heart rate in each of the workloads to be used (the two between 110 beats/min and 150 beats/min) should be plotted against the respective workload on the maximum physical working capacity prediction graph (figure 6.25). The first load is not used in this calculation unless it has exceeded 110 beats/min. A straight line is drawn through the two points and extended to that participant's predicted maximum heart rate.

The point at which the diagonal line intersects the horizontal predicted maximum heart rate line represents the maximum working capacity for that participant. A perpendicular line should be dropped from this point to the baseline where the maximum physical workload capacity can be read in kgm/min.

Examples: Plotting the Maximum Physical Working Capacity

The first subject has been given all three workloads according to the previously described directions. The results follow.

Age_ 40 _years   Weight_ 176 _lb   80 _kg

Physical Working Capacity Test

Seat height_ 8 _   Predicted max heart rate_ 180 _bpm

85% of predicted max heart rate _153_ bpm _11.8_ seconds for 30 beats

Workloads		Heart Rates	
1st workload	150kgm	101	2nd min
		105	3rd min
			4th min (if needed)

MAXIMUM PHYSICAL WORKING CAPACITY PREDICTION

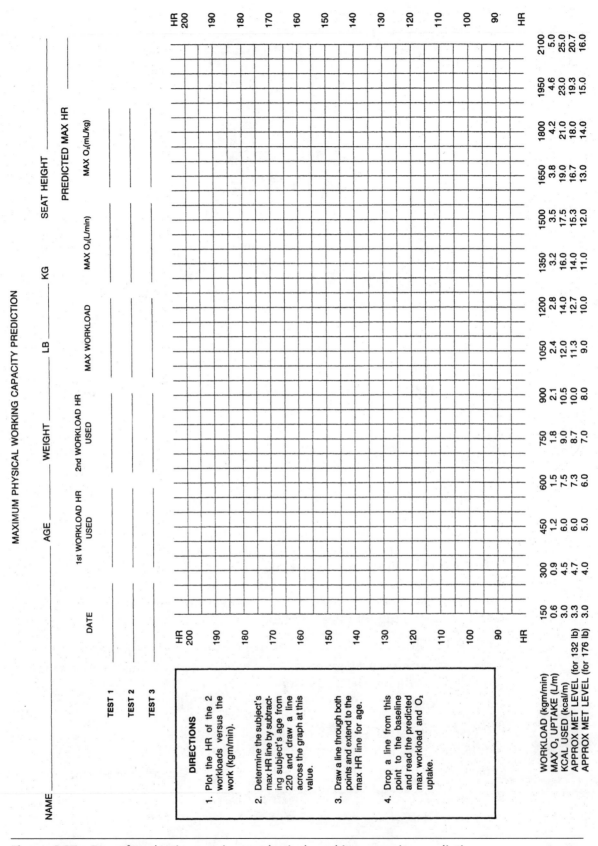

Figure 6.25 Form for plotting maximum physical working capacity prediction.

2nd workload	_300_ kgm	_116_ 2nd min
		_120_ 3rd min
		_____4th min (if needed)
3rd workload	_450_ kgm	_142_ 2nd min
		_145_ 3rd min
		_____4th min (if needed)

The heart rates in the third minute of the second and third workloads are plotted against their respective workloads. This entire calculation is shown in figure 6.26. A line is drawn through these points and extended to the predicted maximum heart rate line as determined by age (i.e., 220 - 40 = 180). A line is dropped to the baseline at the intersection of these two lines, and the predicted maximum workload is determined (i.e., 650 kgm/min). Maximum oxygen uptake can also be predicted from this test. The predicted maximum oxygen uptake in this example is $1.6\ L \cdot min^{-1}$ or 1600 ml. 1600 ml divided by the body weight in kilograms computes to a maximum oxygen uptake in ml/kg ($\dot{V}O_2max$), which is 20 ml of oxygen for every kilogram of body weight in one minute, which is written in the scientific literature as $ml \cdot kg^{-1} \cdot min^{-1}$. This calculation is made easy by the use of table 6.10. Enter weight and $\dot{V}O_2max$ and where the two intersect is the $ml \cdot kg^{-1} \cdot min^{-1}$ value.

A second subject has been given only two workloads because the first workload elicited a heart rate greater than 110 beats/min. The test was given according to the previously described directions. Here are the results.

Age_ 30 _years   Weight_ 121 _lb   _55_ kg

Physical Working Capacity Test

Seat height_ 6 ___   Predicted max heart rate_ 190 _bpm
85% of predicted max heart rate_ 161 _bpm _11.2_ seconds for 30 beats

Workloads		**Heart Rates**
1st workload	150kgm	_109_ 2nd min
		_112_ 3rd min
		_____4th min (if needed)
2nd workload	_300_ kgm	_121_ 2nd min
		_125_ 3rd min
		_____4th min (if needed)

3rd workload not necessary

The heart rate in the final minute of the first and second workloads is plotted against the respective workloads. This entire calculation is shown in figure 6.27.

A line is drawn through these points and extended to the predicted maximum heart-rate line. Where the lines intersect, a perpendicular line is dropped to the baseline. This line indicates a predicted PWC maximum of 1050 kgm/min for this example. This means that, had the subject worked until the maximum heart rate was elicited, he or she would have been cycling at 1050 kgm. The predicted maximum oxygen uptake is $2.4\ L \cdot min^{-1}$. Divided by body weight in kilograms $2.4\ L \cdot min^{-1}$ yields a maximum oxygen uptake of $43.64\ ml \cdot kg^{-1} \cdot min^{-1}$ ($\dot{V}O_2$ divided by weight, or 2400 ml/55 kg). This calculation is made easy by the use of table 6.10.

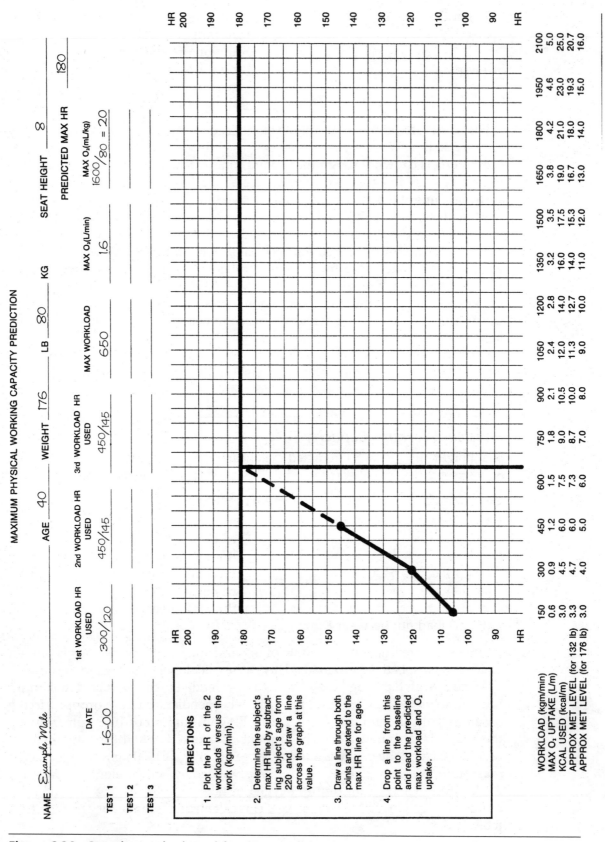

Figure 6.26 Sample graph plotted for three workloads.

152

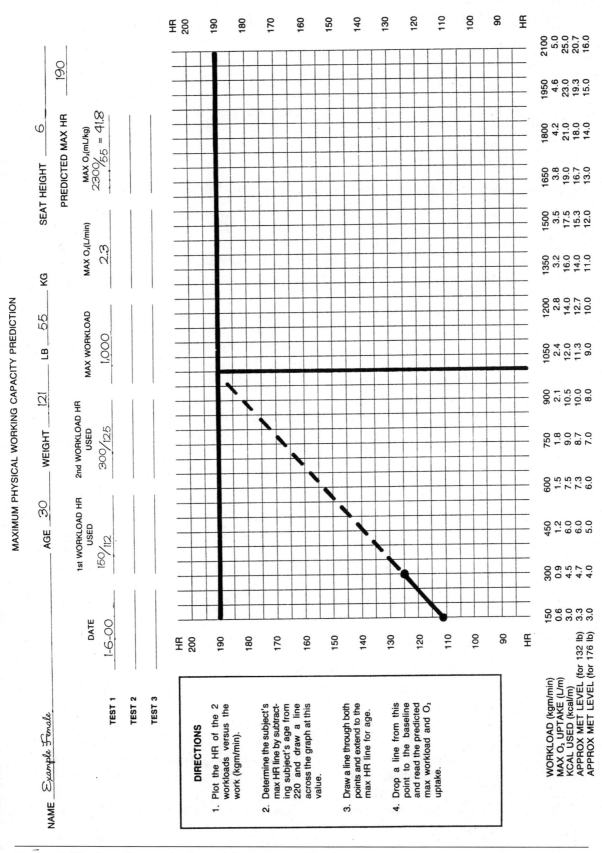

Figure 6.27 Sample graph plotted for two workloads.

Test Interpretation

The YMCA cycle ergometer test provides two measures that are useful in evaluating cardiovascular-respiratory function and working capacity: predicted maximum physical working capacity and predicted maximum oxygen uptake.

Remember that these tests are estimates or predictions of maximal responses and have a greater chance of being in error than would be the case if the participants were to exercise to their actual maximum. Interpretation must therefore be made carefully, and the possibility of poor or incorrect predictions must be understood.

Predicted Maximum Physical Working Capacity (PWC)

The predicted maximum PWC shows the workload at which the heart rate is expected to reach its maximum value. Assuming the test is done correctly, the greatest source of error is the possibility that the age-estimated maximum heart rate is not correct. Research has shown that the maximum heart rate has a wide range of values at any age. If the estimate is too high, maximum PWC will be overestimated; if it is too low, it will be underestimated. Accuracy can be improved if the true maximum heart rate is known. This is sometimes available if the participant has, for some reason, recently taken a stress ECG test. However, regardless of the possible errors, the norm tables are based on 220 minus age. Some individuals know their maximum HR from a graded exercise test given at the hospital. Even if someone claims to know his or her maximum HR, do not use it for this test; use the predicted maximum HR.

The greatest value in using the maximum PWC comes from comparing results before and after a participant enters an exercise program. Substantial improvement can be expected with regular participation in a YMCA exercise program. Data can also be compared to norms presented in appendix B.

Predicted Maximum Oxygen Uptake

The predicted maximum oxygen uptake is an extension of the PWC test. It is useful because so much interest in maximum oxygen uptake is being generated in current scientific and popular literature. As with the maximum PWC, improvement is expected with conditioning, and the results can be compared to available norms.

Assuming that the test is done correctly, the predicted maximum oxygen uptake is subject to the same source of errors as is the predicted maximum PWC, that is, the accuracy of the age-estimated maximum heart rate. There is also a second source of error. The oxygen uptake is calculated from the estimated maximum work rate. The assumption is that everyone expends the same amount of energy and uses the same amount of oxygen at a given work rate (energy expenditure is computed from the volume of oxygen used). The test will underestimate the true maximum for an individual who is very inefficient (expending a disproportionately large amount of energy to perform a given task) and will overestimate the true maximum oxygen uptake for an individual who is very efficient. Participants who are unfamiliar with bicycle exercise tend to be less efficient than those who bicycle regularly.

When actually measuring maximum oxygen uptake, most studies show that maximum oxygen uptake can be improved about 15% to 20%.

General Observations and Interpretation

As noted previously, both the maximum PWC and oxygen uptake can be compared to norms or used to demonstrate training effects; however, both are age dependent.

Use of the energy expenditure data in appendix D is also important in interpreting results. By determining the MET and kilocalorie values from the chart, it is possible to anticipate an individual's response to exercise. According to the energy expenditure table in appendix D, the first example subject's maximum working capacity, which is slightly greater than 8 kcal per minute as estimated by the test, would be the equivalent of cycling approximately 9.4 mph. This energy expenditure is less than the amount of energy needed for chopping wood fast, running 11.5 miles, or engaging in vigorous activity while skin diving. Examples of activities that require an expenditure of approximately 8 kcal/min would be playing tennis or skiing in soft snow. If the vertical lines drawn to intersect the chart axis are dropped at other heart rates, similar comparisons can be made.

No matter how the test results are used, the validity of the interpretations and the usefulness to the participant depend on obtaining high-quality data. The test must be given as described. The bicycle ergometer must be well maintained, which means regular calibration and proper maintenance. The environment must be well controlled, free from both physical and emotional stress. If the tester has any doubts about the results, he or she should test again to be sure.

3-Minute Step Test

When YMCAs need to test large groups of participants at once, the cycle ergometer is impractical. As a substitute, the 3-Minute Step Test can be used very successfully in mass-testing situations. This step test is an excellent cardiorespiratory test not only for mass testing but also as a self-test or as an addition to a test battery. The test requires minimal equipment, and participants can learn to administer it to themselves by counting the carotid or radial pulse; however, when performed as a part of the test battery, it should be done as described here.

Equipment

The following equipment is used for the step test:

1. A 12-in. high, sturdy bench
2. A metronome set at 96 beats/min (Four clicks of the metronome equal one step-up, up, down, down at 24 steps per minute. See the earlier section in this chapter on metronomes, page 143.)
3. A timer for the three minutes and a timer for the recovery (these may be the same)
4. A stethoscope to count recovery heart rate
5. Testing forms to record data

Procedure

Demonstrate the stepping. Face the bench and, in time with the metronome, step one foot up on the bench (first beat), step up with the second foot (second beat), step down with the first foot (third beat), and step down with the other foot (fourth beat). The sequence is alternating feet. It does not matter which foot leads or if the lead foot changes during the test (see figure 6.28). Do not allow the participant to practice, as it will affect the heart rate.

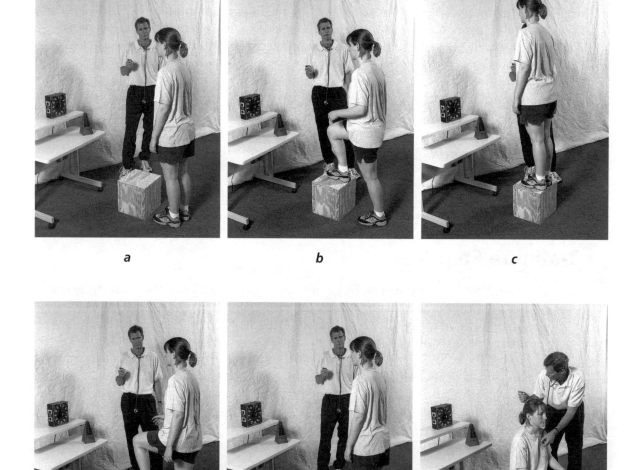

a   b   c

d   e   f

Figure 6.28 Three-minute step test. (a) Starting position; (b) step up; (c) up position; (d) step down; (e) down position; (f) heart rate count.

Explain to the participant both the test and the importance of sitting down quickly at the end of three minutes and remaining still for one minute so that the tester can count the heart rate. Position the participant facing the bench and allow him or her to pick up the beat of the metronome by marking time in place. When the participant starts stepping, start the timer. Check the rhythm and correct if necessary. Inform the participant of the time as it passes by saying "one minute," "two minutes," and so on.

When 20 seconds remain, remind the participant that he or she is to sit down quickly at the end of the stepping and wait for the tester to take the heart rate. Put the stethoscope in your ears and prepare the recovery timer. On the last step it is helpful to say, "Last step-up, up, down, and sit." It might be helpful to turn the metronome off during the last 15 seconds of stepping and count the cadence for the participant until the last step.

When the participant sits down, immediately place the stethoscope on the chest, get the rhythm, and within five seconds, start counting for one full minute. Begin the count on a beat, counting that beat as "zero." The recovery rate count must be started within five seconds or the final heart rate count will be significantly different. (*Note*: Pay close attention to the heart's rhythm, which can change suddenly during recovery. It is easy to lose count.) The one-minute count reflects the heart's rate at the end of stepping as well as the rate of recovery.

The total one-minute heart rate is the score for the test and can be recorded and compared to the norms in the scoring sheets in appendix B or to previous test results if appropriate. Score the total one-minute postexercise heart rate in beats per minute.

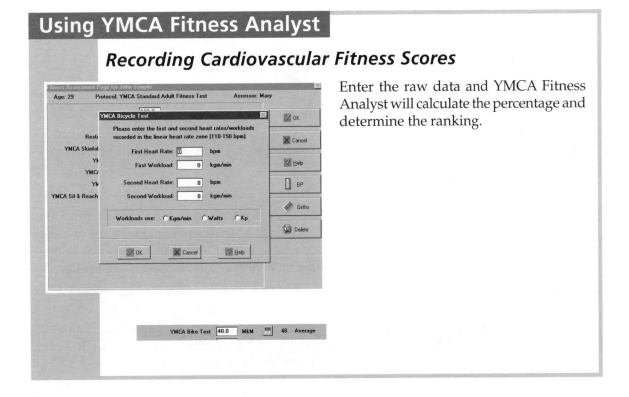

Using YMCA Fitness Analyst

Recording Cardiovascular Fitness Scores

Enter the raw data and YMCA Fitness Analyst will calculate the percentage and determine the ranking.

Tests of Flexibility

Much of the American adult population has low back pain. Often this is related to reduced flexibility of the hip and back because of tightness of the hamstring muscles. Many of these conditions can be improved by following a well-designed program of stretching exercises that increases the flexibility of the hips and back.

Although no one general flexibility test will assess the flexibility of an individual because flexibility is specific to each joint, trunk and hip flexion has been used for the past 40 years as a general test of flexibility. In 1941 Cureton published an article on flexibility that introduced the Trunk-Forward Flexion Test. In the 1950s, Scott and French (1959) modified the trunk flexion test. The development and modification of this flexibility test has a long history, with the last modification developed by Johnson and Nelson in 1979.

YMCA Flexibility Test

The flexibility test presently used in the YMCA Fitness Assessment protocol is the sit-and-reach test. YMCAs may also want to consider using the AAHPERD Older Adult Flexibility Test for their older members.

Test Administration

There is a limited possibility that the subject could strain the back with too vigorous a movement in this test. It is recommended that the test be performed slowly and cautiously.

Equipment

The following equipment is necessary for the flexibility test:

1. A yardstick or tape measure to measure the distance reached, a line drawn (or a piece of tape) on the floor at right angles to the 15-in. mark, with the zero mark toward the participant
2. Tape to keep the measuring instrument in place on the floor and to mark a line
3. Testing forms to record data

An inexpensive flexibility board can be built out of scrap plywood and a short length of a 2' x 4' (see figure 6.29). The board can be easily stored and can conveniently facilitate the administration of this test. In addition, commercially available trunk-flexion instruments are available and can be used successfully.

Procedure

The flexibility test requires a minimum of equipment and can be administered on any floor. Simple equipment to speed up the test can be built as just described. Adequate warm-up and stretching should be done prior to doing this test. Normally the test is given after the cycle ergometer or the step test so that participants are already warmed up; however, additional stretching, especially of the hamstrings, is advised. Participants must also be cautioned against making any fast, jerky movements, which increase the risk of injury.

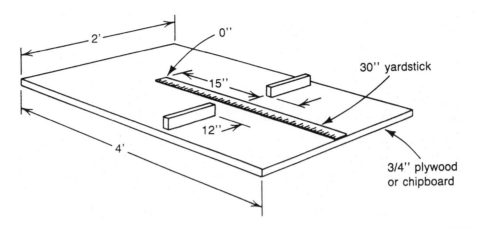

Figure 6.29 Handmade flexibility board.

Place a yardstick on the floor and put a 12- to 15-in. piece of adhesive tape across the yardstick at the 15-in. mark and at right angles to the tape. Have the participant sit with the yardstick between the legs with the 0-in. mark toward the crotch and the knees extended and the legs abducted about 12 in. Shoes should be removed, and the heels of the feet should nearly touch the edge of the taped line. When the individual leans forward down the yardstick, the heels tend to slide forward, so if the participant starts about an inch behind the line, the heels will be in the correct position (see figure 6.30). The 2' x 4' wooden strips on the flexibility board prevents any forward sliding, eliminating time used in trial and error.

With the fingertips in contact with the yardstick, have the participant slowly reach forward with both hands as far as possible on the yardstick, holding this farthest position momentarily. To get the best stretch, the participant should exhale and drop the head between the arms when reaching. Be sure that the participant keeps the hands parallel and does not stretch or lead with one hand. Ensure that the participant's knees are kept straight by gently holding the knees down. Have the participant do three trials, and record the best stretch of the three in inches. Normally the score is recorded to the nearest half-inch, although it could be recorded to the closest one-quarter inch. The norm table records whole-inch divisions.

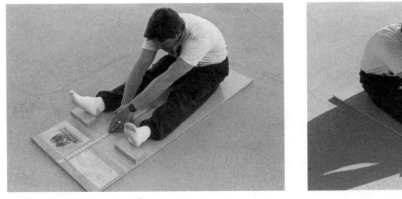
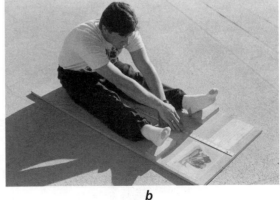

a   *b*

Figure 6.30 Correct position for the flexibility test.

A recent study by Golding showed a significant difference in the scores obtained in the YMCA Flexibility Test and a different version of the sit-and-reach test used in some other test batteries. To use the YMCA's norms the test must be performed as just described.

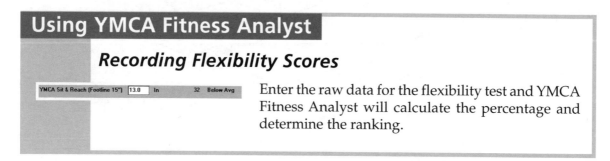

Using YMCA Fitness Analyst

Recording Flexibility Scores

YMCA Sit & Reach (Footline 15") [13.0] In 32 Below Avg

Enter the raw data for the flexibility test and YMCA Fitness Analyst will calculate the percentage and determine the ranking.

AAHPERD Older Adult Flexibility Test

The AAHPERD flexibility test for older adults uses the "box" flexibility test. This test uses a specially made box, which can also be purchased commercially. The box is a cube measuring 12 x 12 x 12 inches. A yardstick is attached to the top of the box with the yardstick projecting over the end of the box so that the projection starts at the 15-in. mark. The subject sits facing the box with the feet (dorsally flexed) against the box under the projecting yardstick. Knees are extended and the subject puts the hands on the yardstick (which is 12 in. above the floor), then slides the hands down the yardstick to the farthest possible point, without jerking. The score is recorded to the nearest half-inch. When testing older adults, extra precaution should be taken against the possibility of injury. When using this test, be sure to use AAHPERD norms.

Tests of Strength and Muscular Endurance

Muscular strength and endurance is an essential component of any physical fitness assessment. Every occupational and recreational activity requires muscular strength. In addition, normal daily living activities such as housework, yardwork, and lifting and carrying require strength.

The testing of strength prior to, during, and after an exercise program is important and desirable. The reasons for measuring strength may be one or more of the following:

1. Assess current strength

2. Identify strength needs

3. Select training regimes

4. Evaluate progress and improvement

5. Evaluate the success of an exercise program in achieving its strength objectives

6. Provide motivation

When testing for strength, the reason for testing should be identified and shared with participants. In addition, the testing procedures as well as muscle groups under study should be explained. The strength tests used should do the following:

1. *Take a minimal amount of time but give a maximal amount of strength information.* The main purpose of any exercise program is the actual exercise; testing is an additional facet of the program that, although desirable, should not detract from the exercise portion of the program.

2. *Identify the muscle groups that are to be evaluated.* Are all muscle groups going to be tested, or just certain groups? What muscles are tested depends on the goals of the program, the amount of testing equipment available, and the time and personnel available to do the testing.

3. *Consider the capability of the tester.* Unless the testing is supervised by a professional, sophisticated testing equipment should be avoided and practical field tests used.

4. *Be simple to administer and interpret.* Field tests like 1 RM (one repetition maximum, the greatest weight that can be moved one time) are relatively easy to administer, understand, and interpret. However, the 1 RM may be too strenuous for the average unfit individual and especially the older adult.

5. *Determine strength for muscle groups that will be exercised in the exercise program.* For example, don't measure grip strength if increasing grip strength is not a goal of the program.

Many individuals exercise for many years. Establishing baseline strength values for the various muscle groups will allow the changes in strength to be tracked over a period of time. Participants who age, who incur joint injuries, or who have joint surgery are often given exercises to rehabilitate the joint by strengthening the muscles surrounding it. If strength testing has been done prior to injury, then the return to preinjury strength can be monitored.

Considerable research has been done on the effect of age on muscular strength. Strength decreases dramatically with age, but current research shows that strength does not have to decrease at the rate it typically does if the muscles are exercised. Physiological age is a better index of age than chronological age. Old age usually means the inability to do the physical tasks that were done when younger. Old age can be defined as the inability to perform physical activities, especially those activities of daily living. This inability often makes the older adult incapable of living independently. Except for injury or pathology, with continued exercise the ability to perform physical activities on one's own does not have to be lost.

In this next section we discuss the limitations and assumptions made in assessing strength and considerations in choosing strength tests; describe the various methods of testing strength; and explain the protocols for the YMCA Bench Press, and Half Sit-Up tests.

Definitions, Limitations, and Assumptions in Strength Assessment

Before we discuss the various methods of measuring strength we must define two terms: muscular strength and muscular endurance.

■ *Muscular strength.* Muscle strength is the maximum pull or push that can be exerted one time by a muscle group. In physiological terms it is the greatest number of muscle fibers that can be voluntarily innervated at one time.

■ *Muscular endurance.* Muscular endurance is the ability of a muscle to contract repeatedly or to hold a contraction for an extended period of time.

Historically, muscular strength has been measured either isometrically or with one maximum isotonic contraction. Muscular endurance has also been measured by the number of repetitions one can do with a given resistance.

In many strength tests such as pull-ups, sit-ups, and push-ups, the purpose is to do as many as possible. Because of the repetitions, these tests are measuring, primarily, muscular endurance. The 1 RM is measuring strength because it determines how much weight can be lifted only once. The greater the resistance, and therefore the fewer the repetitions, the more the test measures strength. The more repetitions, therefore the lighter the resistance, the more muscular endurance is being measured. A continuum from very heavy (measuring strength) to very light (measuring muscular endurance) tests can be performed.

Considerations in Strength Assessment

Many experts and practitioners believe strength should be measured dynamically, that is, with movement. An example would be one maximum dynamic contraction, called 1 RM (or one repetition maximum). Others believe that more reliability can be obtained with a maximum static contraction. A static measure means assessing strength without movement, for example, one maximum pull or push against an immovable resistance. This measure is typically employed with a dynamometer, strain gauge, load cell, or cable tensiometer.

Most physical fitness test batteries include one or two tests of strength or muscular endurance. Historically, most physical fitness tests have used push-ups, chin-ups, and sit-ups to evaluate muscular strength. The Air Force, Navy, Marine Corps, Army, Boy Scouts, 4-H Clubs, and AAHPERD have all used push-ups or chin-ups, or modifications of these, to assess the strength component of physical fitness.

When the YMCA's test battery was first published, one of the strength tests was grip strength. The grip-strength dynamometer was relatively inexpensive and easy to use, easy to interpret, relatively nonstressful, and widely discussed in the literature. Through several years of use, it was noted that the grip strength of participants did not change even though it was obvious that individuals had gained in strength, that is, they were able to do a higher number of repetitions of various strength exercises. The reason for the lack of change detected by the grip strength was that little is done in the average fitness class that improves grip strength.

When the YMCA's test battery was revised, a more valid strength test was needed. Push-ups and chins are commonly used in dozens of physical fitness test batteries. The reason for this is that early strength research showed that a fair relationship exists among elbow flexion, elbow extension, and total strength. This finding motivated test creators to use push-ups (elbow extension) and pull-ups (elbow flexion).

Due to the weight of the body, both of these tests are extremely difficult, resulting in many individuals getting a score of zero. If 10 individuals all receive a score of zero there is no way to distinguish the amount of strength difference among these individuals. Zero is a nondiscriminating score group, in which a large number of people are lumped together into one group. To overcome this limitation some test batteries employ modified push-ups and chins. If elbow flexion and extension are fair indicators of total strength then free weights can be used to lessen the resistance. Instead of chins and push-ups, curls and bench presses could be substituted. The same muscle groups are used but with less resistance. The YMCA decided to use the bench press and the half sit-up as substitutes for grip strength.

YMCA Bench Press Test

In developing the YMCA Bench Press Test as the preferable test of muscular strength, much discussion and trial focused on the selection of the right weight to use. A heavy weight would measure strength but would not discriminate among the strength levels of participants, as there potentially would be too many people unable to perform even one repetition. A light weight would allow for everyone to do the test but would result in a high number of repetitions and be measuring primarily muscular endurance. It was decided that a weight was needed that would result in subjects averaging 15 repetitions. Hopefully, this weight would allow all those tested to be able to do at least one repetition, but not too many would be able to do many repetitions. The test would, therefore, measure both strength and muscular endurance.

Three universities conducted trials on both men and women to determine the weight that would result in an average of 15 repetitions. It was found that a total weight (bar, collars, and weights) of 35 pounds for women and 80 pounds for men gave a mean of 15 repetitions for both groups. This was field tested in YMCAs on 8400 people. Fifteen repetitions proved to be the approximate mean for all age groups and both sexes. It was also determined that with this resistance and this untrained population, body weight was not correlated with the results; therefore, body weight was ignored.

This test has been used in YMCAs since 1985 and has proven to dramatically show changes in strength and muscular endurance in those who exercise regularly.

YMCA Half Sit-Up Test

Because the abdominal musculature in adults becomes weak with disuse, many exercise programs stress abdominal exercise. Many adults want a flat abdomen. For this reason an abdominal strength test was deemed necessary. The obvious test was sit-ups. Full sit-ups have been criticized and have been considered, by most, as a contraindicated exercise. This resulted because of the hip flexors that are also used in the full sit-up. One of the major hip flexors is the psoas muscle which originates on the five lumbar vertebra. When the hips flex, the origin of the psoas tries to pull the lumbar vertebra forward, exaggerating the "lordosis effect" of the low back. This pulling of the lumbar vertebra can aggravate individuals with low back pain. In the full sit-up the abdominal muscles are supposed to prevent this "tilting" forward of the pelvic girdle, but if the abdominal muscles are weak the tilting does occur.

Fitness instructors today don't recommend doing leg lifts, for the same reasons as the criticism of the full sit-up. The cantilevering effect on the pelvic girdle in leg lifts causes the psoas muscle to pull the lumbar vertebra forward, which is undesirable because it can aggravate the low back, especially in individuals who have low back problems. Although the prime movers in leg lifts are the hip flexors, leg lifts are done to exercise the abdominals. In the leg lifts the abdominals are stabilizers of the pelvic girdle preventing it from tilting forward and keeping the low back in contact with the floor, thereby exercising the abdominals isometrically. Because precaution to keep the low back on the floor is often not stressed, and leg lift exercises typically allow the forward tilting of the pelvis to occur, the exercise is no longer recommended.

At the time the YMCA's fitness test battery was being constructed there were no valid and reliable abdominal tests except the full sit-up with the feet held down and the hands clasped behind the head. The test was used for 20 years, although some individuals with known back problems were told not to do this test. However, although it was explained that the full sit-up was used only for testing and not for exercise, many resisted doing the test. In response, the YMCA has developed a half sit-up test (more like the exercise used in classes), which has been validated and proven reliable.

In half sit-ups (also called abdominal crunches, partial sit-ups, and partial curl-ups) the spine is flexed 30°; the half sit-up does not recruit the hip flexors and places less stress on the lower back. Performing the half sit-up with the feet unsupported and the knees flexed maximizes abdominal muscle activity and minimizes hip flexor activity (Godfrey et al. 1977; Halpern and Bleck 1979). Different researchers have reported that abdominal muscle activity is maximized by different degrees of knee flexion. On the basis of electromyographic (EMG) studies, the optimal angle of the knees has been variously reported to be 45° (Flint 1965), 65° (Walters and Partridge 1956), and 90° (LaBan et al. 1965).

Largely because of the stress they place on the lower back, full sit-ups have been replaced by half sit-ups in exercise programs. Despite this fact, full sit-up tests are sometimes still used to assess abdominal strength and endurance, probably because of ease of administration and the availability of standardized protocols and established norms. For the same reasons that half sit-ups have replaced full sit-ups in most exercise programs, the YMCA decided that it would be valuable to develop a standard test of abdominal muscular strength and endurance employing half sit-ups. Two types of half sit-up protocols have been proposed: one requiring unlimited repetitions (Faulkner et al. 1989; Jette et al. 1984) and one requiring timed one-minute protocols (Macfarlane 1993; Reebok 1991; Robertson and Magnusdottir 1987). A review of this research and subsequent study by Diener et al. (1995) resulted in a new protocol adopted by the YMCA.

The angle of the knees and the height of the curl are critical. Raising the body to 30° is necessary to maximally involve the abdominals. The sliding of the fingers forward 3½ in. ensures that the upper body is curled up 30°. (See abdominal crunch test protocol.)

Strength Testing Methods and Equipment

A number of strength testing modalities may be employed, including the following:

- 1 RM (repetition maximum)
- 10 RM
- Dynamometer
- Cable tensiometer
- Load cells or strain gauges
- Strength exercises

1 RM (Repetition Maximum)

The greatest weight that can be moved one time is called 1 RM. The weight is determined by trial and error. The 1 RM can be determined for any muscle group and is a dynamic strength measurement because movement (one repetition) takes place. Many training protocols call for a percentage of the 1 RM. Because of the trial-and-error methods, 1 RM is time consuming to determine, although it has been shown to be a reliable test.

10 RM

The RM can be preceded by any number and is the maximum number of repetitions that can be done with a particular weight. 10 RM is the weight that can be lifted just 10 times. In reading strength literature percentages the 10 RM is often encountered. Multiple RMs is a measurement of muscular endurance because it involves repetitions.

Dynamometer

A dynamometer is a spring scale against which the strength of a muscle is measured. The most commonly available dynamometers are the grip dynamometers and the back and leg dynamometer. This latter measuring device consists of a metal or wood base plate, a chain, a belt, a handle, and the dynamometer.

The subject stands on the base plate to which the dynamometer is attached. The dynamometer is then either attached to a handle for back strength, or to a belt for leg strength. The subject exerts maximum pull, which the dynamometer registers in lb or kg. Because practically no movement is involved, the dynamometer is considered a measure of isometric or static strength.

The criticism of the back and leg dynamometer is that multiple joints are used (plantar flexion, knee extension, hip extension, spine extension) and body weight becomes a major factor. Individuals tend to "surfboard," that is, lean back. Huge weights can be recorded, which cannot be duplicated when muscle groups are isolated.

The grip strength dynamometer discussed earlier measures the strength of the grip. An attachment for some grip strength dynamometers (push-and-pull attachment) allows for shoulder abduction and adduction to be measured. Spring devices traditionally need constant calibration because as springs are used, they become more and more flexible and inaccurate.

Cable Tensiometer

The cable tensiometer was developed for the aircraft industry during World War II. It measures the pounds of tension on a flexible cable. The tensiometer has a movable riser that slightly kinks the cable. The tighter the cable, the more pressure is needed to kink it; this pressure is read on an arbitrary scale calibrated into pounds. It was discovered that this instrument could be readily adapted for strength testing. In strength testing the principle of the cable tensiometer is similar to the dynamometer. A muscle group pulls on the cable and the tension on the cable is measured. This system is more flexible than the dynamometer, and the strength of all muscle groups can be easily measured with the help of a strength-testing table. Special harnesses and aircraft cable of different lengths can be made to accommodate all body movements. Elaborate strength testing tables have been built to facilitate these measurements. No movement is required, so the angle of the joint during testing must be clearly established and used in strength studies. In the 1960s Harrison Clarke conducted numerous studies describing a strength table, specifying the methods of testing each muscle group, and determining the best angle to be used at each joint. The criteria for selecting the angle of the joint were the point where strength was greatest, where the angle provided the best test-retest reliability, or where the angle was most comfortable for the subject.

Load Cells or Strain Gauges

The load cell or strain gauge method is identical to the cable tensiometer except that instead of using a tensiometer to kink the cable, the load cell or strain gauge replaces the tensiometer and actually measures, electrically, the force applied to the cable. Both the load cell and strain gauge produce an electrical output that can be recorded and can produce a strength curve on a graph, or create a digital readout. These devices are light in weight, easily used, and easily calibrated. The measurement is also isometric. Like the tensiometer, the load cell or strain gauge method is also used in conjunction with a table, cables, and harnesses.

Strength Exercises

The easiest and most practical method of measuring either the strength or muscular endurance of any muscle group is to do an exercise that uses the muscle group.

How many push-ups, pull-ups, or sit-ups can the participant accomplish? Or how many bench presses, curls, pullovers, etc., can he or she do? Individuals can be tested before beginning a strength program and again 12 or 16 weeks later. Retesting is an excellent way of keeping a record of strength gains. Calisthenics are limiting, however, because body weight does not change and repetitions often become high, measuring more muscular endurance than strength.

This method of strength testing can be done with free weights, the Universal Gym, Nautilus, or any of the strength training machines. Each muscle group can be tested for 1 RM or 6 RM, or any number desired. Because fewer repetitions reflect testing more of the strength component, and more repetitions reflect testing more of the muscular endurance component, strength testing on equipment might be efficiently done with 3 RM. Each major muscle group can be isolated and the 3 RM for that muscle group recorded. Retest each muscle group at 8 or 12 weeks and plot strength changes.

Measuring the number of a specific strength exercise provides an indication of dynamic strength, which gives instant feedback on strength acquisition. For most individuals, it is the most practical measurement of strength.

Other Strength Measuring Instruments

Many other good strength measuring instruments are available, among them Cybex, Orthotron, Chattex, Iso-B100, and the Jackson strain gauge, just to name a few. The Cybex has been widely used in strength research, as it permits the measurement of muscle strength, power, and endurance. Many of these instruments are found in research laboratories or physical therapy offices but are not routinely used by strength trainers.

YMCA Bench Press Test

The YMCA has developed a standard method of measuring dynamic strength, through the use of a common strength exercise—the barbell chest press.

Equipment

The following equipment is necessary to administer the bench press test:

1. 35-lb barbell (women); 80-lb barbell (men)
2. Metronome set for 60 beats/min
3. Conventional bench used for pressing weights or a similar bench approximately 12-in. wide, 50-in. long, and 17- to 20-in. high (A lower bench should be built for shorter individuals.)
4. Testing forms to record data

Procedure

Have the participant lie on the bench in a supine (face-up) position, with the knees bent and the feet on the floor. Hand the barbell to the participant, who has elbows flexed and palms up (down position). The participant should grip the bar with the hands approximately shoulder-width apart (see figure 6.31a). Have the participant then press the barbell upward to extend the elbows fully (see figure 6.31b). After each extension the participant should return the barbell to the original down position. The metronome sets the rhythm, with each click representing a movement up or down (60 beats/min). Encourage the participants to breathe regularly and not to strain during the test. Holding one's breath while exerting force can cause what is known as the Valsalva maneuver, a dramatic increase in intrathoracic pressure and blood pressure, which could cause one to black out.

A word about the use of the metronome is necessary here. Without a ticking metronome the participant will typically complete a few repetitions, then rest for a few seconds and then continue. The participant may start and stop several times, with the rest period in between getting longer and longer. Those who are experienced in

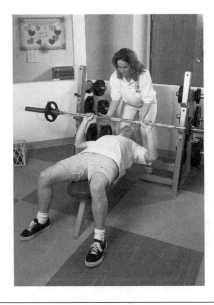 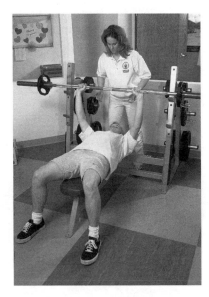

Figure 6.31 Bench press test. (a) Starting position; (b) extension.

strength testing will recognize this scenario. When the individual stops and the tester asks if he or she is finished, the answer is almost always "No, I can do some more." The participant will then continue, starting and stopping several times. To eliminate this habit, the metronome was introduced. The tester should instruct the participant to do as many repetitions as possible or to continue until he or she can no longer keep pace with the metronome. A speed of 60 beats/min was established by observing and timing the speed of bench pressing on a large group of non-weight lifters. The metronome is used only to keep the rhythm. A little faster or slower pace is satisfactory as long as the pace is maintained.

Scoring

Score the number of successful repetitions. The test is terminated when the participant is unable to reach full extension of the elbows or he or she breaks cadence and cannot keep up with the rhythm of the metronome.

For safety, at least one spotter should be present during the test. If a single spotter is physically unable to catch the weight, two spotters should be present, one at each end of the barbell. Record the results and compare them to the norm table for the age and gender of the subject.

YMCA Half Sit-Up Test

As previously mentioned, muscular endurance is difficult to test due to the number of different muscles and muscle groups involved. Another problem is the subjective end point of most muscular endurance tests, which is somewhat dependent on motivation. Controlling the technique of execution used during testing is another difficulty. The one-minute timed sit-up test was initially selected for the following reasons. First, it is fairly representative of general muscular endurance. Second, the test measures one of the most important muscle groups of the middle-aged individual. Third, it is fairly standardized with respect to technique. And, last, the one-minute time period reduces the influence of motivation.

As mentioned earlier, the use of full sit-ups as an exercise is controversial, and it is not being recommended that full sit-ups be given in an exercise class. Half sit-ups, or crunches, exercise the abdominals better and do not strain the lower back. The half sit-up test reliably measures abdominal muscle strength and endurance more safely.

Equipment

The following equipment is used to conduct the half sit-up test:

1. A stopwatch or clock with a sweep second hand to time the crunches.
2. A mat. Although not absolutely necessary, a 48-in. x 26-in. plywood board can be covered with a neoprene pad. (Padding makes the test more comfortable for the subject. However, the test can be given on any floor surface.)
3. Four 6-in. strips of self-adherent Velcro, placed rough-side up, perpendicular to the body. The strips are placed 3.5 in. apart.
4. Testing forms to record data.

Procedure

The participant lies supine with knees bent at right angles and hands pronated and the fingertips on the first strip of Velcro. The tester instructs the participant to maintain the shoulders in a relaxed position (neither depressed nor elevated). Compliance with this instruction must be verified visually by the tester. At a "go" signal from the timer, the participant performs as many correct crunches as possible within a one-minute period, with a partner maintaining the count. The subject should flex the spine (curl up) so that the fingertips of each hand reach the second strip of Velcro, then return to the starting position. The shoulders must be returned to touch the mat, but the head need not touch. Score the number of repetitions in one minute. (*Caution*: The participant should breathe easily during the exercise so as not to invoke the Valsalva maneuver.)

Summary of Half Sit-Up Study

1. The one-minute half sit-up test showed high test-retest reliability ($r = 0.98$).

2. The inter-tester reliability of the one-minute half sit-up test is high ($r = 0.76$).

3. The one-minute half sit-up test showed a moderately high correlation with the one-minute full sit-up test ($r = 0.66$).

Using YMCA Fitness Analyst

Recording Muscular Strength Scores

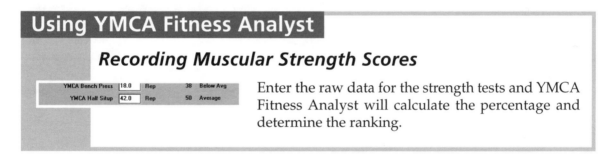

Enter the raw data for the strength tests and YMCA Fitness Analyst will calculate the percentage and determine the ranking.

Chapter 7

Planning and Administering Fitness Testing

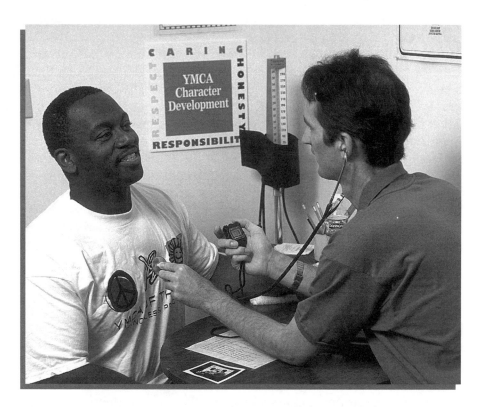

Once the fitness director becomes knowledgeable about fitness testing and familiar with the YMCA Fitness Assessment protocol, he or she must understand how to implement a testing program at the local YMCA. Factors such as how fitness testing fits into the overall programming and membership goals of the YMCA must be considered. Will all new members be offered a free fitness assessment, as is the practice in some Ys, or will assessment be made available to anyone for an additional fee? Will training of additional staff be necessary to assist with the testing? How will appointments for testing be handled? Implementation of a fitness testing program also includes administering the tests in a consistent and reliable manner, interpreting and explaining the test results to members, and using the results to prescribe meaningful and useful individual exercise programs. Testing, to be accurate and beneficial for members, takes considerable preparation. Careful planning is required to make the testing procedure operate smoothly and safely. Test details must be considered to ensure that the results are as accurate as possible. Administrators must make certain that test participants are informed and prepared; they must also have an understanding of what to do with the results once they are obtained.

To Test or Not?

Fitness assessments can serve as a valuable tool in assisting and guiding YMCA members in their exercise experiences. Providing useful information based on scientifically sound measurements can help people exercise in a safe, effective manner and develop the foundation for a lifetime of physical activity. For many, testing and evaluation prior to starting an exercise program and periodically thereafter is considered an important way to assess current fitness levels, identify training needs, evaluate progress, and provide ongoing motivation and education.

YMCA fitness directors need to remember, however, that not everyone wants or even needs to undergo a fitness assessment prior to beginning a physical activity routine. The experience of a fitness test can be unpleasant and demotivating for overweight and unconditioned individuals; most likely their scores will be low and the tests may produce muscle soreness. Rather than subject individuals to such an experience, it may be more valuable to start someone on a low-level fitness program of walking and/or other moderate activity to increase their fitness level slowly and gradually. Once the person becomes more comfortable with activity and develops some conditioning, assessments may become appropriate, and the fitness director can recommend a more specific exercise prescription. The fitness director's goal should be to use a variety of methods to increase the physical activity levels of members, so they may ultimately lead healthier lives. The professional director should use good judgment in recommending whether or not a fitness assessment is appropriate for any member.

Guidelines for Administering Fitness Assessments

Administering fitness assessments accurately requires a certain amount of skill, which can only be developed through practice. Attending the five-day YMCA of the USA Fitness Specialist training course is a good place to start developing that skill, but the course alone does not adequately prepare participants to administer the tests. A common mistake is for YMCAs to allow tests to be given before the competency of the tester is proven. After completion of the YMCA certification course and prior to working with members, staff should participate in practice testing sessions with other staff members to refine their testing skills as well as their ability to interpret test scores.

A key factor in ensuring the validity and reliability of fitness tests is adhering to consistent guidelines whenever the tests are administered. This consistency will help ensure that the tests are given the same way every time, that participants are given the preliminary information that they need, and that staff all follow the same procedures. Following are some suggested guidelines for conducting fitness assessments at your YMCA.

1. Establish a site for fitness testing that is private, contains all the equipment needed, and does not have to be set up each time a test is given. The recommended room size for a fitness testing area is 9 ft x 12 ft. This room can also be the area for storage of records and a place to consult with members during the test interpretation session. Keep in mind that for valid and reliable $\dot{V}O_2$max values, the testing area should be maintained at a temperature between 68° and 74° Fahrenheit and at a humidity level of 50 percent.

2. Establish emergency procedures for fitness testing particular to the site or location of the test area.

3. Make sure that the equipment required to conduct the fitness testing battery is available and functioning properly:

- Cycle ergometer—The model manufactured by Monark is recommended
- Step bench—12 in. in height
- Skinfold calipers—Either a Lange or Harpenden caliper is recommended
- 80-lb and 35-lb barbells for men and women, respectively
- Flat exercise bench for bench press test
- Exercise mat and Velcro strips for half sit-up test
- Yardstick, tape measure, or flexibility measuring device
- Metronome (or an audiotape of a metronome)
- Stethoscope
- Sphygmomanometer
- Scale for height and weight
- Stop watch
- Timer

4. Give the participants written instructions on how to prepare for their fitness assessment, including the following:

- Wear comfortable, loose fitting clothing or regular exercise attire.
- Avoid eating or drinking (e.g., coffee, tea, or soda) for at least three hours before the test.
- Avoid using alcohol and tobacco for at least eight hours before the test.
- Avoid exercising on the day of the test.
- Get a good night's sleep the evening before the test.
- Complete and bring all required forms to the testing session.

5. Establish a screening procedure of test participants that should include a PAR-Q form, an informed consent form for fitness testing, a health history questionnaire, and medical clearance if needed. Appropriate forms can be found in appendix A and in the Fitness Analyst software program.

6. Establish a schedule of when testing will be offered, based on the availability of the Fitness Specialist, and set up a procedure for appointments to be made and necessary information to be given to participants.

Using YMCA Fitness Analyst

Scheduling Appointments

The Comprehensive Edition of YMCA Fitness Analyst includes a Staff and Member Scheduling Page. This page allows you to keep track of any appointments you have, noting what the appointments are for and, if payments are due, the amount of the payment and whether the payment was made. You can link each of the member appointments to the corresponding member folders so you can bring members' records up quickly for review. The software also lets you create a To Do list that allows you to prioritize your tasks.

7. Conduct the tests in the recommended order to ensure their accuracy, as follows:

- Begin by allowing participants to rest for at least five minutes to recover from activity involved in getting to the YMCA (e.g., traffic, getting children to child care, etc.).
- Conduct the resting measurements of heart rate and blood pressure.
- Conduct the body composition skinfold test.
- Conduct the cardiorespiratory (cycle ergometer or 3-minute step) test.
- After a suitable rest period, conduct the flexibility test.
- Conduct two muscle strength and endurance tests.
- Have the participant cool down upon completion of the tests.

8. Schedule an appointment to review and interpret the test results, as soon as possible after the completion of tests. At this time, you should also be prepared to discuss and recommend an exercise prescription for the participant.

9. When retesting participants, the tests should be repeated at the same time of day, using the exact same procedures. Consistency in retesting will help ensure the accuracy of the test results for comparison purposes.

Using YMCA Fitness Analyst

Creating a Fitness Test Protocol

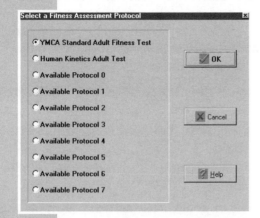

If you would like to use other tests in addition to the standard YMCA tests, YMCA Fitness Analyst provides you with several test protocols that can be customized or helps you to select individual tests to create your own. Descriptions of each of the tests are available through the Help function.

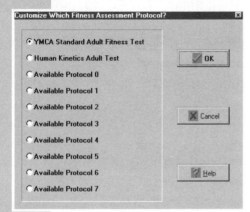

Here's one example of how a set test protocol can be customized.

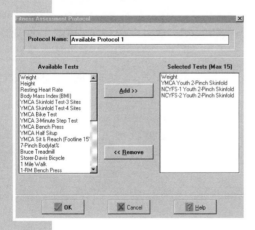

YMCA Fitness Analyst makes it simple to add to or substitute tests already in your protocol. The software will then change all the test-result recording pages accordingly.

Interpretation of Fitness Assessment Results

Interpreting the results of a member's fitness assessment is the critical first step in developing a personalized exercise routine. The YMCA fitness director must be skilled in understanding test results and translating that information into an exercise prescription that is appropriate for the member. The fitness director should do the following when conducting a test interpretation session with a member who has undergone a fitness assessment:

- Assess the member's current physical fitness status based on test scores in comparison to the appropriate norm table for his or her gender and age.
- Discuss the member's personal goals, both short and long term, related to health and physical activity.
- Discuss the member's areas of interest, focusing on those activities that he or she enjoys and is more likely to maintain.
- Discuss roadblocks to achievement of goals, such as work and/or family obligations, travel, environmental conditions, and accessibility to a center like the YMCA in which to exercise.
- Establish realistic short- and long-term goals based on the member's interests, activities, and potential obstacles that must be overcome.
- Get the member started in a program designed to meet his or her personal goals.

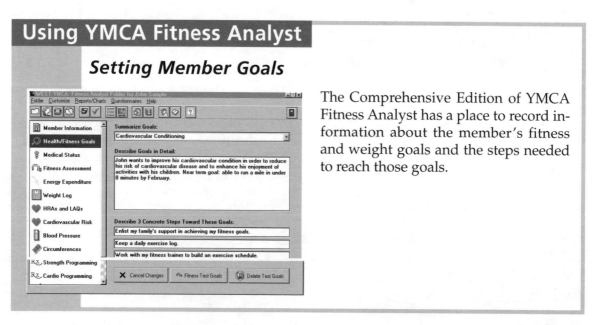

Using YMCA Fitness Analyst

Setting Member Goals

The Comprehensive Edition of YMCA Fitness Analyst has a place to record information about the member's fitness and weight goals and the steps needed to reach those goals.

The fitness director should schedule a private, one-on-one session to interpret the test results with the member and begin a dialogue to develop an individualized fitness plan. Normative information on each test should be shared with the member, with a careful and concise explanation of where the individual ranks, according to his or her gender and age, for each fitness measurement. Presenting the test results to the member in a manner that is positive and motivating requires some sensitivity on the part of the staff. The following should always be considered:

▪ Be aware of the psychological and medical implications that a participant may derive from the interpretation. Do not consciously or unconsciously make a medical diagnosis. If you are uncertain how to answer a question, it is best to acknowledge that you are not sure, but you will find the information and relay it to the participant later.

▪ Present the information in a way that is understandable, useful, and specific to the participant.

▪ Utilize all sources of information when interpreting the test results, including the participant's health history, exercise history, and personal observations.

▪ Provide test results and interpretation as soon after the assessment as possible. Participants are usually anxious to hear how they did and what their scores mean.

▪ Thoroughly explain the norm charts to the individual, showing how he or she ranks according to gender and age for each test. Remember to point out that the ranking is based on comparison to others his or her age who have taken the same tests.

A thorough understanding of fitness principles and how the test scores provide indications of various measures of one's fitness level is crucial in conducting a meaningful interpretation session. Like administering the actual tests, the counseling and sharing skills needed for this session can be gained and polished through practice. Staff may want to conduct role-playing sessions with each other to become more comfortable in test interpretation and exercise prescription.

Using YMCA Fitness Analyst

Printing Reports

YMCA Fitness Analyst provides a number of reports that you can share with participants. They usually enjoy having a written record and explanation of their test results that they can take home. You can customize these reports with the name of the participant and the name and address of your YMCA. Here are some of the reports available that could help you during the test interpretation session:

The Comprehensive Report of Findings includes information from all data entered from fitness testing, questionnaires, health-risk assessments, and analyses performed.

YMCA

103 E Main, Springfield, USA
PH: 208-555-1212 FAX: 208-555-1212

Comprehensive Report of Findings

Prepared for   Prepared By
John Sample   **YMCA Assessor**

This report is designed to give you a complete overview of all of the analyses we have performed to date. It summarizes your measured performance or health risk indices and provides feedback to help you understand where you are doing well and where you may need improvement. The report will also expand your understanding of health issues and help you and your trainer plan your personal program of health and fitness enhancement.

This introductory text can be edited in any way you choose. You may enter whatever information is necessary to meet the overall needs of your client.

continued

Using YMCA Fitness Analyst, *continued*

The Member Goal Report is a printed record of the member's stated goals and the steps he or she will take to meet them.

The Lifestyle Assessment Report explains the implications of the member's responses to the YMCA Lifestyle Assessment Questionnaire. It also includes information on how the member can improve lifestyle habits.

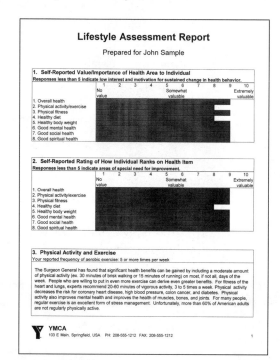

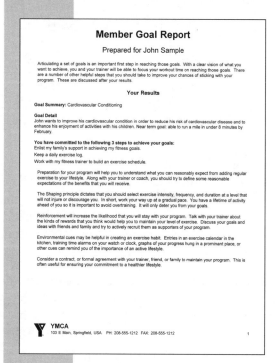

The Framingham Heart Risk Report summarizes the member's risk of developing cardiovascular heart disease (CHD). It also includes the American Heart Association's tips for reducing CHD risk.

Guidelines for Exercise Prescription

Conducting and then interpreting the results of a fitness assessment are the first two steps in the process of engaging an individual in physical activity. The third step is using that information to design an exercise program for the person that will meet his or her needs and goals and that he or she will be able to follow and enjoy for a long time. *Exercise prescription* is a common term in the field of exercise science used to describe the process by a trained, certified professional with special knowledge of fitness and exercise who develops a personalized plan for someone to follow. When used appropriately by fitness professionals, *exercise prescription* is a good term, which is defined by the American College of Sports Medicine as: "the process whereby a person's recommended regimen of physical activity is designed in a systematic and individualized manner" (1995). The fitness director should remember, however, that providing information to members on appropriate levels of exercise is something that health and fitness professionals have been doing for years, long before the term *exercise prescription* came into vogue. For years physical educators developed exercise programs, routines, and regimes and devised progression and training schedules for athletes as well as healthy children and adults. The track and field or swimming coach was trained to know which exercise and training protocols to use with her or his athletes. The progression, adaptation, intensity, and duration were often determined by observation of participants and their performance levels.

Like the term *contraindicated exercise*, the term *exercise prescription* was initially used in the cardiac rehabilitation field before it was adopted by mainstream fitness. Physicians gave postcoronary patients a prescription that indicated how often, how long, and at what intensity the patient should work, or to warn which exercises were contraindicated. The coronary rehabilitation exercise leader made sure that the patient did what was prescribed. Likewise, it is common for a physical therapist to work with his or her patient under a prescription from the physician for a particular rehabilitative purpose. Given the current acceptance of the term to describe a specified program of physical activity, *exercise prescription* is now being used by exercise leaders for individuals in a variety of physical fitness programs.

It is appropriate to use the term *exercise prescription* when addressing principles such as mode of exercise, duration, frequency, and intensity for an apparently healthy individual. Exercise leaders should understand, however, that they are not providing the same type of exercise prescription that might be given by a physician and followed by a physical therapist or cardiac rehabilitation specialist. Fitness directors need to understand the limits of their scope of practice and expertise and advise participants accordingly.

Once a person's fitness capacity has been determined through assessment, health status known through questionnaires and/or clearances, and interests and goals expressed, an individualized exercise prescription can be given. To be effective, a prescription must be based on all three of these factors. The exercise leader can then develop specific guidelines for the intensity, duration, frequency, type, and progression of exercise, the integral components of a sound exercise prescription.

Because the reasons for exercising can vary greatly among individuals of all different fitness levels, the need for precision in prescribing exercise will also vary. Performance athletes and persons limited by disease may require careful and precise prescription; average, apparently healthy adults, however, rarely need precision, and general principles of exercise and training are usually adequate. Most such people will select activities that they enjoy or that allow them to have social and recreational interaction. The important point to remember is that the same principles of training apply to everyone. Modifications are usually associated with the absence or presence of medical contraindications, types of activities to be avoided, the initial level of fitness, the intensity of participation, and the rate of improvement expected.

The following text focuses on the five primary factors that should be considered in developing fitness prescriptions for apparently healthy adults: frequency, intensity, duration, mode of activity, and rate of progression. These five factors are discussed in terms of the three primary components of physical fitness: cardiorespiratory conditioning, muscle strength and endurance, and flexibility. This information is based on the American College of Sports Medicine's position paper on exercise prescription, which includes recommendations concerning the quantity and quality of exercise training for healthy adults (1998).

Cardiorespiratory Conditioning

1. *Frequency of training*: Three to five days per week.

2. *Intensity*: 55/65% to 90% of maximal heart rate. It should be noted that exercise of low and moderate intensity may provide important health benefits and may result in increased levels of fitness in sedentary and low-fit individuals.

3. *Duration of training*: Twenty to 60 minutes of continuous aerobic activity. The actual length of time spent exercising aerobically is dependent on the relative intensity level of the activity. For example, activities of a lower intensity should be conducted over a longer period of time, particularly early on in one's training.

4. *Mode of activity*: An appropriate modality for developing cardiorespiratory fitness is any activity that uses the large muscle groups, can be maintained at submaximal levels continuously, and is rhythmical in nature. Examples are walking, jogging, running, bicycling, swimming, aerobic dancing, machine-based stair climbing, rowing, and cross-country skiing. It should be noted that activities such as walking, jogging, or cycling are particularly good activities to start out with as one begins an exercise program.

5. *Rate of progression*: Because of the ability of the body to adapt to the stresses placed upon it (referred to as the *training effect*), individuals are able to gradually increase the total work they can do over time. With cardiovascular exercise, increasing the work performed can be achieved by increasing the intensity of the exercise, the duration of the exercise, or by some combination of the two. The most significant training effects are typically observed during the first six to eight weeks of an exercise program. One's exercise prescription can be adjusted as these conditioning effects occur. The extent of the adjustment depends on the individual involved and the performance of the individual during exercise sessions.

Muscle Strength and Endurance

1. *Frequency of training*: Minimum of two days per week.
2. *Intensity*: Moderate-intensity resistance training, sufficient to develop and maintain lean body tissue.
3. *Duration of training*: One set of 8 to 12 repetitions of each exercise.
4. *Mode of activity*: Eight to 10 exercises that train the major muscle groups of the body.
5. *Training guidelines*:
   - Adhere to the specific techniques for performing each exercise.
   - Exercise to the point of momentary muscular fatigue.
   - Perform each exercise through a full range of motion.
   - Exercise antagonist muscle groups.
   - Perform both lifting and lowering movements in a controlled manner.
   - Be conscious of not holding the breath while strength training. Be sure to exhale when exerting force.

Flexibility

1. *Frequency of training*: Minimum of two to three days a week.
2. *Intensity*: Stretch to a position of mild discomfort.
3. *Duration of training*: Ten to 30 seconds for each stretch.
4. *Mode of activity*: Stretching should include appropriate static and/or dynamic techniques, with an emphasis on the low back and hamstring area due to the prevalence of low back pain.
5. *Repetitions*: Two to six for each stretch.

Use a form such as the sample YMCA Exercise Prescription Form shown in figure 7.1 to help organize and record the individualized exercise prescriptions you create for members.

Developing an Appropriate Exercise Prescription

The fitness director should remember that desirable fitness outcomes for members can be attained with exercise programs that vary considerably in terms of mode, frequency, intensity, and duration. In addition, some individuals achieve a faster and/or greater rate of improvement than others. For example, members who have been relatively sedentary for years should be counseled to progress more slowly. They should begin exercising at a level that they can successfully complete and then gradually increase the amount of work they perform. This slow progression not only reduces the potential for injury, but it also ensures appropriate adaptations in previously unused or underused muscles. Conversely, active individuals may progress more rapidly, so as not to become frustrated, as they are more ready to be challenged physically. The skill of the fitness director will be in recognizing how individuals are adapting to an exercise routine and making necessary and appropriate adjustments to prescriptions.

YMCA Exercise Prescription Form

Warm-Up
Purpose: To gradually elevate the heart rate and increase body temperature by engaging in 5 – 10 minutes of low-intensity activity.

Cardiovascular Fitness
Purpose: To improve one's cardiorespiratory system by continuous, rhythmic, and vigorous exercise, for 20 – 30 minutes, 3 times a week.

Frequency – Days a week of exercise: Mon. Tues. Wed. Thur. Fri. Sat. Sun.

Intensity – % of heart rate: Max. HR – Age x 55% to 90% = Training HR range

Duration – No. of minutes per session: 10–20   20–30   30–45

Mode – Select activity:

Cool-Down
Purpose: To gradually decrease the heart rate by slowing the intensity and pace of the activity for 5 – 10 minutes.

Muscle Strength and Endurance
Purpose: To develop muscular strength and endurance using various calisthenic and weight training exercises, for 10 – 20 minutes.

Exercises:

Muscle: _____   Exercise:_____   Resistance: _____   Repetitions: _____

Muscle: _____   Exercise:_____   Resistance: _____   Repetitions: _____

Muscle: _____   Exercise:_____   Resistance: _____   Repetitions: _____

Muscle: _____   Exercise:_____   Resistance: _____   Repetitions: _____

Muscle: _____   Exercise:_____   Resistance: _____   Repetitions: _____

Muscle: _____   Exercise:_____   Resistance: _____   Repetitions: _____

Muscle: _____   Exercise:_____   Resistance: _____   Repetitions: _____

Flexibility
Purpose: To stretch the major muscles and joints using static stretching techniques, for 5–10 minutes.

Exercises: _____

Figure 7.1   YMCA Exercise Prescription Form.

Using YMCA Fitness Analyst

Programming Exercise

YMCA Fitness Analyst provides you with a number of resources for exercise prescription.

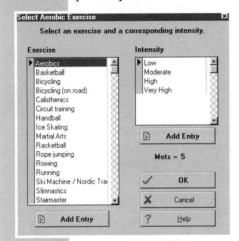

The Cardio Programming page allows you to select from a number of types of aerobic exercise.

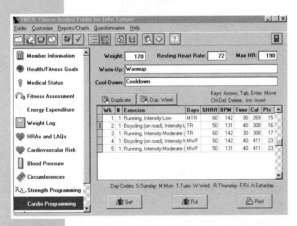

Once you select the exercise, YMCA Fitness Analyst will estimate the number of calories the exercise will burn, based on the MET value of the exercise and the member's weight. If you fill in the percentage of heart-rate reserve desired during the exercise, it also will calculate what the target heart rate should be.

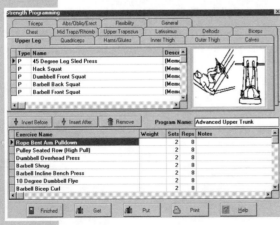

The Strength Programming page allows you to design strength training programs for members by selecting appropriate exercises from the strength exercise library.

continued

Using YMCA Fitness Analyst, *continued*

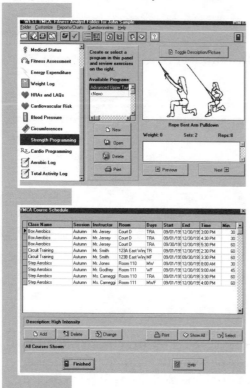

Each exercise has a written description and is accompanied by a drawing. You can print out this information for the member.

Finally, you can build a database of all your Y's fitness courses and use it to create a customized list of YMCA courses for each member, depending on his or exercise needs.

A Prescription for Life

Physical activity can be a valuable tool in improving the health and fitness levels of YMCA members. To assist them in receiving the maximum benefits of exercise, the fitness director must analyze their personal needs, interests, health status, and current fitness level. Using that information, a personal plan for exercise can be established that will meet the member's unique requirements. Remember that all exercise prescriptions should closely adhere to the primary prescription variables for a sound exercise regimen. With periodic adjustments as appropriate, you will help give each member a prescription for a lifetime of health and fitness.

Using YMCA Fitness Analyst

Tracking Member Participation

The Comprehensive Edition of YMCA Fitness Analyst has three aids for tracking ongoing member participation in your fitness program: the Aerobic Log, Energy Expenditure, and Total Activity Log pages.

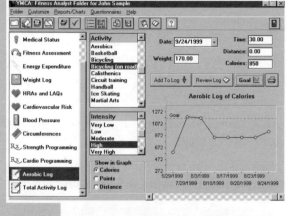

The Aerobic Log page allows you to record completed aerobic activities. It will estimate the number of calories burned during the activity, based on the type of activity, its intensity, the participant's weight, and the length of time the activity was performed. In addition, it will add the activity to a graph of calories expended that also shows the goal level of calorie expenditure.

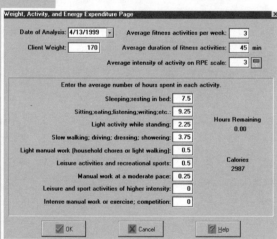

The Energy Expenditure page can be used to estimate a member's total daily caloric expenditure, including any exercise he or she performs on a regular basis.

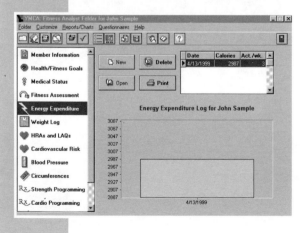

The estimation can be repeated and will be graphed automatically.

continued

Using YMCA Fitness Analyst, *continued*

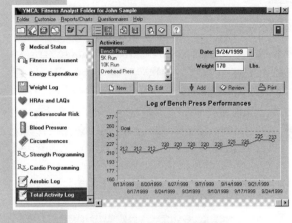

The Total Activity Log page helps you keep track of all of a member's physical activities, whether they are formal exercises or home and garden chores.

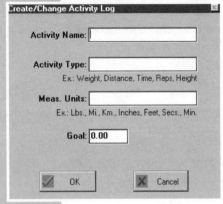

You can add any type of activity and set a goal to reach for that activity.

The record of the activity and its relation to the goal is automatically graphed with each entry.

Using YMCA Fitness Analyst

Educating Members About Fitness

Once you have the results of testing and assessment, you may be able to see where members need help in developing a healthier lifestyle. To guide them you can print out any of 20 different Health and Fitness Education Reports (developed by Dr. David Nieman, Appalachian State University) on topics such as nutrition, body composition, and designing an exercise program. These reports can be edited if needed to better fit your situation.

Nutrition: The Prudent Diet

For all individuals, whether physically active or inactive, a "prudent diet" is recommended for general health and prevention of disease. This diet is advocated for fitness enthusiasts (those exercising three to five days per week, 20 to 30 minutes per session) and nearly all athletes, including those in most individual, dual, and team sports, and power events (weightlifting, track and field). For the competitive endurance athlete (who trains more than 90 minutes a day in such sports as running, swimming, and cycling), several adaptations beyond the prudent diet are beneficial, including a higher percentage of carbohydrate, less fat, and more water. There are seven major dietary guidelines:

1. Eat a Variety of Foods
More than 40 different nutrients classified into six groups (protein, carbohydrate, fat, vitamin, mineral, and water) are needed for good health. These nutrients should come from a variety of foods--not from a few highly fortified foods or supplements--because no single food can supply all of these nutrients in the necessary amounts. Supplements of some nutrients, when taken regularly in large amounts, can be harmful. As a general rule, most Americans don't need the supplements for good health.

Diet variety is probably the single most important nutrition principle. Grains and cereals should form the basis of each meal, supplemented with liberal servings of vegetables and fruit and low-fat servings of dairy and meat products. Typical serving sizes are one slice of bread or one-half cup of pasta; one-half cup of cooked vegetables; one medium apple, banana, or other fruit; one cup of milk or yogurt; and two to three ounces of cooked lean meat, poultry, or fish.

2. Balance the Food You Eat With Physical Activity to Maintain or Improve Your Weight
Being overweight is common in the United States and it is linked with high blood pressure, heart disease, stroke, diabetes, certain cancers, arthritis, and other types of illness. A healthy weight can be maintained by being physically active and consuming a variety of foods low in calories and fat--such as fruits, vegetables, whole grains, non-fat dairy products, and baked fish or poultry.

Body Composition

Interest in the measurement of body composition has grown tremendously during the last 20 years, largely because of its relationship to both health and athletic performance. Recent scientific data have linked obesity with coronary heart disease, several types of cancer, stroke, diabetes, osteoarthritis, high blood cholesterol, and high blood pressure.

Body weight can be divided into fat and fat-free weight. The fat-free weight is primarily muscle, bone, and water. Body composition is often defined as the ratio of fat to fat-free weight.

There are several methods used to measure body composition such as skinfold pinch tests, bioelectrical impedance, and underwater weighing. These methods result in an estimation of percent body fat. Percent body fat, which is the percent of total weight represented by fat weight, is the preferred index used to evaluate a person's body composition. If the percent body fat is known, then a desirable weight can be determined.

Target Weight vs Ideal Weight
Desirable weight is also known as Target Weight. Target weight is calculated as lean body weight (the body weight with no fat) plus some desired percentage of fat. Target weight, a better term than ideal weight, is the weight an individual is aiming to attain.

Height-weight tables provide weight ranges that are recommended for a certain height, but they provide only a rough estimate of one's healthy body weight. People vary widely in their fat-free weight, such that muscular and athletic individuals are usually defined as "overweight" when using the height-weight tables despite having low amounts of body fat. At the same time, those with small amounts of muscle and bone can often be designated as "underweight" when in actuality they may be carrying too much body fat. Ideal weight brings up the question of "ideal for what?" Ideal weight for a marathoner is different from that for a professional football player or for an Olympic gymnast. Marathon runners may wish to have 10% to 12% fat (as many marathon runners are), whereas weight lifters or football players may prefer to be 15% to 20% fat.

For these reasons, it is recommended that concerned individuals have their body fat measured at a reputable health and fitness facility to gain a true picture of their percentage

Selecting an Aerobic Exercise

Selection of the appropriate type of aerobic exercise is central to the long-term success of an exercise program. Most studies have shown that if frequency, intensity, and duration of training are similar, the cardiorespiratory training outcomes are independent of the mode of aerobic activity. In other words, if different people cycle, swim, or run for five days a week, 30 minutes a session at a similar intensity (e.g., 75 percent of the maximum rate), after 10 to 15 weeks, improvement in heart and lung fitness should be comparable.

It should be noted, however, that some aerobic activities like rowing and swimming also confer considerable musculoskeletal benefits, giving more of a "total fitness" benefit when compared to running or cycling, for example.

Any aerobic activity mode, such as jogging, walking, cycling, stair climbing, swimming, or rowing, should be selected on the basis of individual interest; time and facility availability; personal goals and objectives; and fitness level. Choose primary and secondary aerobic activities that you can fit into your schedule without creating undue stress and inconvenience.

"Lack of time" is the major obstacle individuals list for not continuing exercise programs. To improve compliance, some people like the socialization, competitiveness, and pleasure of various dual and team sports. Many sports can develop aerobic and musculoskeletal fitness, improving compliance for those who enjoy this type of exercise. Others enjoy various work activities such as splitting wood or shoveling dirt, feeling that while overall fitness is being improved, they are also accomplishing a worthwhile task.

National surveys show that the most popular fitness activity continues to be walking, followed by swimming, bicycle riding, exercising with equipment, basketball, and aerobic dancing. Moderate-intensity activities of longer duration are being promoted more and more by fitness leaders, because these types of activities are more acceptable to the masses, increasing the likelihood of a permanent change in lifestyle. Physical activities such as brisk walking result in low rates of musculoskeletal injury and have the potential to lower blood pressure, improve the lipid profile, reduce body fat, enhance mental well-being, and reduce the risk of coronary heart disease and cancer. Walking has been found to have a higher compliance rate than other physical activities because it can

Exercise and Aging

During the last century, dramatic improvements in life expectancy have been achieved in many countries worldwide. In the United States, for example, life expectancy (or the number of years a newborn baby can expect to live) has increased from 47 to nearly 76 years during the 1900s, and is expected to exceed 82 years by the year 2050.

In simple terms, the baby boomers are getting old, a phenomenon many experts call the "age wave." In 1900, for example, only 40 percent of Americans lived beyond age 65, while in 1990 this proportion had risen to 80 percent.

The central issue raised by increasing longevity is that of quality of life. The National Center for Health Statistics has estimated that 15 percent of the average American's life is spent in an "unhealthy" state (that is, impaired by disease, disabilities, and/or injuries). Among those reaching age 65, five of their remaining 17 to 18 years, on average, will be unhealthy ones.

Health habits have a strong influence on both life expectancy and quality of life during old age. Dr. Lester Breslow, in his famous study of over 6000 people in the San Francisco Bay area, showed a dramatic difference in death rate between those people who followed seven simple health habits (never smoked, moderate or no alcohol consumption, daily breakfast, no snacking, seven to eight hours of sleep per night, regular exercise, ideal weight) and those who did not. Those who followed all seven health habits were estimated to live nine years longer and suffer less disability than those who did not practice any of them. In other words, healthful living appears not only to promote longevity but also to increase the chance of having the physical ability to enjoy life to its fullest in later years.

A key ingredient to healthy aging, according to many gerontologists, is regular physical activity. Of all age groups, the elderly have the most to gain by being active, including the potential for decreased risk of heart disease, cancer, high blood pressure, depression, bone fractures, and diabetes, as well as improved body composition, fitness, longevity, ability to perform personal care activities, and management of arthritis. Yet national surveys indicate that only about one-third of the elderly exercise regularly, which is less than any other age group.

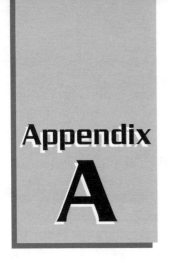

Appendix A

Health Screening, Medical Clearance, and Informed Consent Forms

The following forms can be reproduced and used as needed for your YMCA classes. The screening forms should be administered when participants enter a program or begin membership, and retaken when their health status changes.

Form I—Health Screen Form (PAR-Q & YOU)

Form I is the Physical Activity Readiness Questionnaire developed by the Canadian Society for Exercise Physiology. It asks for general information about the participant's physical condition. Individuals should be instructed to follow the recommendations based on their answers prior to participating in YMCA fitness testing or exercise programs.

Forms II and IIA—Medical Clearance Form and Testing/Exercise Program Description

The Medical Clearance Form is used by the participant's physician to report any restrictions that should be placed on the participant during fitness testing or exercise programs. The physician should see both Form II and Form IIA, which describes generally the YMCA fitness testing and exercise programs and the risks associated with each.

Form III—Informed Consent for Fitness Testing

The Informed Consent for Fitness Testing form ensures that the participant is aware of the risks involved in the fitness testing procedures. It documents that a description of the testing procedures has been read and that all questions concerning those procedures have been answered satisfactorily.

Form IV—Informed Consent for Exercise Participation

The Informed Consent for Exercise Participation form ensures that the participant is aware of the risks involved in exercise. It documents that the description of the exercise program has been read and all questions concerning the exercise program have been answered to the participant's satisfaction.

When and How to Use the Forms

The Health Screen Form (Form I) should be completed before a participant starts any program, even if it is just an education class. The information obtained in this form is valuable for educating participants on potential health and cardio-vascular risk. Note that Form I is not intended to be a medical exam but simply a means of obtaining key health information.

If a potential participant requires medical clearance, use Form II. It allows a physician to indicate that he or she thinks the individual is capable of participating in the Y's exercise programs. Form IIA provides a description of the YMCA exercise programs for the doctor.

The informed consent forms (Forms III and IV) are designed to notify participants of the inherent risks of fitness testing and exercise programs. Form III, Informed Consent for Fitness Testing, should be given to any person registering for a fitness test. It should be read and signed before testing starts. Form IV, Informed Consent for Exercise Participation, should be given to any participant in a supervised exercise program. It should be read and signed before exercise starts.

Determine Your Readiness to Participate in Physical Activity

Complete the following questionnaire (reprinted from the Canadian Society for Exercise Physiology 1994) to help you determine your readiness to begin or intensify a physical activity program.

Physical Activity Readiness
Questionnaire – PAR-Q
(revised 1994)

PAR - Q & YOU

(A Questionnaire for People Aged 15 to 69)

Regular physical activity is fun and healthy, and increasingly more people are starting to become more active every day. Being more active is very safe for most people. However, some people should check with their doctor before they start becoming much more physically active.

If you are planning to become much more physically active than you are now, start by answering the seven questions in the box below. If you are between the ages of 15 and 69, the PAR-Q will tell you if you should check with your doctor before you start. If you are over 69 years of age, and you are not used to being very active, check with your doctor.

Common sense is your best guide when you answer these questions. Please read the questions carefully and answer each one honestly: check YES or NO.

YES	NO	
☐	☐	1. Has your doctor ever said that you have a heart condition <u>and</u> that you should only do physical activity recommended by a doctor?
☐	☐	2. Do you feel pain in your chest when you do physical activity?
☐	☐	3. In the past month, have you had chest pain when you were not doing physical activity?
☐	☐	4. Do you lose your balance because of dizziness or do you ever lose consciousness?
☐	☐	5. Do you have a bone or joint problem that could be made worse by a change in your physical activity?
☐	☐	6. Is your doctor currently prescribing drugs (for example, water pills) for your blood pressure or heart condition?
☐	☐	7. Do you know of <u>any other reason</u> why you should not do physical activity?

If you answered

YES to one or more questions

Talk with your doctor by phone or in person BEFORE you start becoming much more physically active or BEFORE you have a fitness appraisal. Tell your doctor about the PAR-Q and which questions you answered YES.

- You may be able to do any activity you want—as long as you start slowly and build up gradually. Or, you may need to restrict your activities to those which are safe for you. Talk with your doctor about the kinds of activities you wish to participate in and follow his/her advice.
- Find out which community programs are safe and helpful for you.

NO to all questions

If you answered NO honestly to <u>all</u> PAR-Q questions, you can be reasonably sure that you can:
- start becoming much more physically active—begin slowly and build up gradually. This is the safest and easiest way to go.
- take part in a fitness appraisal—this is an excellent way to determine your basic fitness so that you can plan the best way for you to live actively.

DELAY BECOMING MUCH MORE ACTIVE:
- if you are not feeling well because of a temporary illness such as a cold or a fever—wait until you feel better; or
- if you are or may be pregnant—talk to your doctor before you start becoming more active.

Please note: If your health changes so that you then answer YES to any of the above questions, tell your fitness or health professional. Ask whether you should change your physical activity plan.

<u>Informed Use of the PAR-Q:</u> The Canadian Society for Exercise Physiology, Health Canada, and their agents assume no liability for persons who undertake physical activity, and if in doubt after completing this questionnaire, consult your doctor prior to physical activity.

You are encouraged to copy the PAR-Q but only if you use the entire form

NOTE: If the PAR-Q is being given to a person before he or she participates in a physical activity program or a fitness appraisal, this section may be used for legal or administrative purposes.

I have read, understood and completed this questionnaire. Any questions I had were answered to my full satisfaction.

NAME _____

SIGNATURE _____   DATE _____

SIGNATURE OF PARENT _____   WITNESS _____
or GUARDIAN (for participants under the age of majority)

©Canadian Society for Exercise Physiology   *Supported by:*   🍁 Health Santé
Société canadienne de physiologie de l'exercice   CANADA   Canada Canada

Reprinted from the 1994 revised version of the Physical Activity Readiness Questionnaire (PAR-Q and YOU). The PAR-Q and YOU is a copyrighted, pre-exercise screen owned by the Canadian Society for Exercise Physiology.

Form II
Medical Clearance Form

Dear Doctor:

_____ has applied for enrollment in the fitness testing and/
name of applicant
or exercise programs at the YMCA. The fitness testing program involves a submaximal test for cardiorespiratory fitness, body composition analysis, flexibility test, and muscular strength and endurance tests. The exercise programs are designed to start easy and become progressively more difficult over a period of time. A more detailed description of the testing and exercise programs is attached in Form IIA. All fitness tests and exercise programs will be administered by qualified personnel trained in conducting exercise tests and exercise programs.

By completing the form below, however, you are not assuming any responsibility for our administration of the fitness testing and/or exercise programs. If you know of any medical or other reasons why participation in the fitness testing and/or exercise programs by the applicant would be unwise, please indicate so on this form.

If you have any questions about the YMCA fitness testing and/or exercise programs, please call.

Report of Physician

_____ I know of no reason why the applicant may not participate.

_____ I believe the applicant can participate, but I urge caution because

_____

_____

_____ The applicant should not engage in the following activities:

_____

_____

_____ I recommend that the applicant NOT participate.

Physician signature _____ Date _____

Name (printed)_____

Address _____ Telephone _____

City and State _____ Zip _____

Form IIA
Description of Fitness Testing and Exercise Programs

Dear Doctor:

The YMCA fitness testing and/or exercise programs for which the participant has applied are described as follows:

Fitness testing—The purpose of the fitness testing programs is to evaluate cardiorespiratory fitness, body composition, flexibility, and muscular strength and endurance. The cardiorespiratory fitness test involves a submaximal test that may include a bench step test, a cycle ergometer test, or a 1-mile walk for best time test. Body composition is analyzed by taking several skinfold measures to calculate percentage of body fat. Flexibility is determined by the sit-and-reach test. Muscular strength and upper-body endurance may be evaluated by the 1-minute, bent-knee half sit-up test and the bench press test.

Exercise programs—The purpose of the exercise programs is to develop and maintain cardiorespiratory fitness, body composition, flexibility, and muscular strength and endurance. A specific exercise plan will be given to the participant based on needs and interests and your recommendations. All exercise programs include warm-up, exercise at target heart rate, and cool-down (except for muscular strength and endurance training, in which target heart rate is not a factor). The programs may involve walking, jogging, swimming, or cycling (outdoor and stationary); participation in exercise fitness, rhythmic aerobic exercise, or choreographed fitness classes; or calisthenics or strength training. All programs are designed to place a gradually increasing workload on the body in order to improve overall fitness and muscular strength. The rate of progression is regulated by exercise target heart rate and/or perceived effort of exercise.

In both the fitness testing and exercise programs, the reaction of the cardiorespiratory system cannot be predicted with complete accuracy. There is a risk of certain changes that might occur during or following exercise. These changes might include abnormalities of blood pressure and/or heart rate. YMCA exercise instructors are certified in CPR, and emergency procedures are posted in the exercise facility.

In addition to your medical approval and recommendations, the participant will be asked to sign informed consent forms that explain the risks of fitness testing and exercise participation before the programs are initiated.

Form III
Informed Consent for Fitness Testing

Name _____
(please print)

The purpose of the fitness testing program is to evaluate cardiorespiratory fitness, body composition, flexibility, and muscular strength and endurance. The cardiorespiratory fitness test involves a submaximal test that may include a bench step test, a cycle ergometer test, or a 1-mile walk test. Body composition is analyzed by taking several skinfold measures to calculate percentage of body fat. Flexibility is determined by the sit-and-reach test. Muscular strength and upper-body endurance may be evaluated by the 1-minute, bent-knee half sit-up test and the bench press test.

I understand that I am responsible for monitoring my own condition throughout the tests, and should any unusual symptoms occur, I will cease my participation and inform the instructor of the symptoms.

In signing this consent form, I affirm that I have read this form in its entirety and that I understand the description of the tests and their components. I also affirm that my questions regarding the fitness testing program have been answered to my satisfaction.

In the event that a medical clearance must be obtained prior to my participation in the fitness testing program, I agree to consult my physician and obtain written permission from my physician prior to the commencement of any fitness tests.

Also, in consideration for being allowed to participate in the fitness testing program, I agree to assume the risk of such testing, and further agree to hold harmless the YMCA and its staff members conducting such testing from any and all claims, suits, losses, or related causes of action for damages, including, but not limited to, such claims that may result from my injury or death, accidental or otherwise, during, or arising in any way from, the testing program.

_____ Date _____
(Signature of participant)

_____ Date _____
(Person administering tests)

Form IV
Informed Consent for Exercise Participation

I desire to engage voluntarily in the YMCA exercise program in order to attempt to improve my physical fitness. I understand that the activities are designed to place a gradually increasing workload on the cardiorespiratory system and to thereby attempt to improve its function. The reaction of the cardiorespiratory system to such activities can't be predicted with complete accuracy. There is a risk of certain changes that might occur during or following the exercise. These changes might include abnormalities of blood pressure or heart rate.

I understand that the purpose of the exercise program is to develop and maintain cardiorespiratory fitness, body composition, flexibility, and muscular strength and endurance. A specific exercise plan will be given to me, based on my needs and interests and my doctor's recommendations. All exercise programs include warm-up, exercise at target heart rate, and cool-down. The programs may involve walking, jogging, swimming, or cycling (outdoor and stationary); participation in exercise fitness, rhythmic aerobic exercise, or choreographed fitness classes; or calisthenics or strength training. All programs are designed to place a gradually increasing workload on the body in order to improve overall fitness. The rate of progression is regulated by exercise target heart rate and perceived effort of exercise.

I understand that I am responsible for monitoring my own condition throughout the exercise program and should any unusual symptoms occur, I will cease my participation and inform the instructor of the symptoms.

In signing this consent form, I affirm that I have read this form in its entirety and that I understand the nature of the exercise program. I also affirm that my questions regarding the exercise program have been answered to my satisfaction.

In the event that a medical clearance must be obtained prior to my participation in the exercise program, I agree to consult my physician and obtain written permission from my physician prior to the commencement of any exercise program.

Also, in consideration for being allowed to participate in the YMCA exercise program, I agree to assume the risk of such exercise, and further agree to hold harmless the YMCA and its staff members conducting the exercise program from any and all claims, suits, losses, or related causes of action for damages, including, but not limited to, such claims that may result from my injury or death, accidental or otherwise, during, or arising in any way from, the exercise program.

_____   Date _____
(Signature of participant)

Please print:

Name _____   Date of birth _____

Address _____   Telephone _____

Name of personal physician _____

Physician's address _____

Physician's phone _____

Limitations and medications _____

_____

Appendix

B Scoring Sheets

YMCA Fitness Assessment

Score Sheet—Men

Name _____ Date _____

Time _____

Age _____ years   Weight _____ lb _____ kg   Height _____ in.

Resting Blood Pressure _____/_____ mmHg   Resting Heart Rate _____ bpm

---

1. SKINFOLDS

Chest	_____	mm
Abdomen	_____	mm
Ilium	_____	mm
Axilla	_____	mm
Scapula	_____	mm
Tricep	_____	mm
Thigh	_____	mm

2. PERCENT FAT

Sum of 4		Sum of 3	
Abdomen	_____	Abdomen	_____
Ilium	_____	Ilium	_____
Tricep	_____	Tricep	_____
Thigh	_____	Sum	_____
Sum	_____		

Percent fat _____ %   Percent fat _____ %

3. TARGET WEIGHT (16% fat) _____ lb

4. PHYSICAL WORK CAPACITY TEST

Seat Height _____ Predicted Max Heart Rate _____ bpm

85% of Predicted Max Heart Rate _____ bpm _____ Seconds for 30 Beats

Workloads

1st Workload 150 kgm

2nd Workload _____ kgm

3rd Workload _____ kgm

Heart Rates

_____ 2nd min
_____ 3rd min
_____ 4th min (if needed)
_____ 2nd min
_____ 3rd min
_____ 4th min (if needed)
_____ 2nd min
_____ 3rd min
_____ 4th min (if needed)

Transfer above results to the PWC graph and compute.

5. FLEXIBILITY

Trunk Flexion _____ in.

6. MUSCULAR STRENGTH & ENDURANCE

Bench Press (80 lb) _____ reps
1-Minute Timed Half Sit-Ups _____ reps

Transfer results to the Physical Fitness Evaluation Profile and the Body Composition Profile.

YMCA Fitness Assessment

Score Sheet—Women

Name _____   Date _____

Time _____

Age _____ years   Weight _____ lb _____ kg   Height _____ in.

Resting Blood Pressure _____/_____ mmHg   Resting Heart Rate _____ bpm

_____

1. Skinfolds

   Chest   _____ mm

   Abdomen _____ mm

   Ilium   _____ mm

   Axilla   _____ mm

   Scapula   _____ mm

   Tricep   _____ mm

   Thigh   _____ mm

2. Percent fat

Sum of 4		Sum of 3	
Abdomen	_____	Abdomen	_____
Ilium	_____	Ilium	_____
Tricep	_____	Tricep	_____
Thigh	_____	Sum	_____
Sum	_____		
Percent fat	_____ %	Percent fat	_____ %

3. Target weight (23% fat) _____ lb

4. Physical Work Capacity Test

   Seat Height _____ Predicted Max Heart Rate _____ bpm

   85% of Predicted Max Heart Rate _____ bpm _____ Seconds for 30 Beats

Workloads	Heart Rates	
1st Workload 150 kgm	_____	2nd min
	_____	3rd min
	_____	4th min (if needed)
2nd Workload _____ kgm	_____	2nd min
	_____	3rd min
	_____	4th min (if needed)
3rd Workload _____ kgm	_____	2nd min
	_____	3rd min
	_____	4th min (if needed)

Transfer above results to the PWC graph and compute.

5. FLEXIBILITY

   Trunk Flexion _____ in.

6. MUSCULAR STRENGTH & ENDURANCE

   Bench Press (35 lb)   _____ reps

   1-Minute Timed Half Sit-Ups   _____ reps

Transfer results to the Physical Fitness Evaluation Profile and the Body Composition Profile.

YMCA of the USA
Physical Fitness Evaluation Profile

Norms—Men 18-25

Name _____ Dates: T1 _____ T2 _____ T3 _____

Rating	% ranking	Resting HR	% fat	3-min step	PWC max (kgm)	Max V̇O2 (mL/kg)	Flexibility	Bench press	Half sit-ups
Excellent	100 95 90	40 51 54	3 5 7	50 71 76	3390 2365 2100	100 75 65	28 23 22	64 49 44	99 83 77
Good	85 80 75	57 58 59	8 9 10	79 82 84	1945 1835 1750	60 56 53	21 20 20	41 37 34	72 66 61
Above average	70 65 60	61 63 65	11 11 12	88 90 93	1670 1595 1530	50 49 48	19 18 18	33 30 29	57 54 52
Average	55 50 45	66 67 69	13 14 15	95 97 100	1460 1405 1355	45 44 43	17 17 16	28 26 24	49 46 43
Below average	40 35 30	70 71 72	16 17 18	102 105 107	1310 1265 1215	42 39 38	15 15 14	22 21 20	41 40 37
Poor	25 20 15	74 77 78	19 20 21	111 114 119	1165 1110 1060	36 35 32	13 13 12	17 16 13	35 33 29
Very poor	10 5 0	82 87 103	23 27 35	124 132 157	980 880 645	30 26 20	11 9 2	10 5 0	27 23 14

Actual Scores T1 _____ _____ _____ _____ _____ _____ _____ _____

  T2 _____ _____ _____ _____ _____ _____ _____ _____

  T3 _____ _____ _____ _____ _____ _____ _____ _____

	T1	T2	T3
Actual Weight	_____	_____	_____
Target Weight	_____	_____	_____
Blood Pressure	___/___	___/___	___/___

YMCA of the USA
Physical Fitness Evaluation Profile

Norms—Men 26-35

Name _____ Dates: T1 _____ T2 _____ T3 _____

Rating	% ranking	Resting HR	% fat	3-min step	PWC max (kgm)	Max V̇O2 (mL/kg)	Flexibility	Bench press	Half sit-ups
Excellent	100 95 90	36 50 53	4 8 10	51 70 76	3300 2280 1980	95 66 60	28 22 21	61 48 41	80 68 62
Good	85 80 75	55 57 59	11 12 13	79 83 85	1845 1740 1660	55 52 50	19 19 19	37 33 30	58 56 53
Above average	70 65 60	61 62 63	14 15 16	88 91 94	1580 1520 1470	48 45 44	17 17 17	29 28 26	52 46 44
Average	55 50 45	65 66 67	17 18 19	96 100 102	1415 1360 1310	42 40 39	16 15 15	24 22 21	41 38 37
Below average	40 35 30	69 70 71	20 21 22	104 108 110	1265 1215 1170	38 37 34	14 14 13	20 19 17	36 34 33
Poor	25 20 15	74 77 78	23 24 26	114 118 121	1115 1055 995	33 32 30	12 11 11	16 13 12	32 30 26
Very poor	10 5 0	81 85 102	27 29 38	126 134 161	935 795 600	27 24 15	9 7 2	9 4 0	21 17 7

Actual Scores T1 ____ ____ ____ ____ ____ ____ ____ ____

T2 ____ ____ ____ ____ ____ ____ ____ ____

T3 ____ ____ ____ ____ ____ ____ ____ ____

	T1	T2	T3
Actual Weight	_____	_____	_____
Target Weight	_____	_____	_____
Blood Pressure	___/___	___/___	___/___

YMCA of the USA
Physical Fitness Evaluation Profile

Norms—Men 36-45

Name _____ Dates: T1 _____ T2 _____ T3 _____

Rating	% ranking	Resting HR	% fat	3-min step	PWC max (kgm)	Max V̇O2 (mL/kg)	Flexibility	Bench press	Half sit-ups
Excellent	100	37	5	49	3080	90	28	55	79
	95	51	11	70	2060	61	22	41	65
	90	55	13	76	1815	55	21	36	60
Good	85	58	15	80	1720	49	19	32	57
	80	59	16	84	1625	47	19	29	52
	75	60	17	88	1550	45	18	26	48
Above average	70	62	18	92	1480	43	17	25	45
	65	63	19	95	1405	41	17	24	44
	60	64	20	98	1360	40	16	22	43
Average	55	66	21	100	1315	38	15	21	39
	50	68	21	101	1270	37	15	20	36
	45	69	22	105	1225	36	15	18	33
Below average	40	70	23	108	1180	35	13	17	32
	35	71	24	111	1135	33	13	16	31
	30	72	25	113	1090	31	13	14	29
Poor	25	75	26	116	1045	30	11	12	28
	20	78	27	119	1005	29	11	10	25
	15	80	28	124	935	27	9	9	24
Very poor	10	83	29	130	845	24	7	6	21
	5	87	31	138	725	21	5	2	13
	0	101	39	163	560	14	1	0	6

Actual Scores T1 _____ _____ _____ _____ _____ _____ _____ _____

T2 _____ _____ _____ _____ _____ _____ _____ _____

T3 _____ _____ _____ _____ _____ _____ _____ _____

	T1	T2	T3
Actual Weight	_____	_____	_____
Target Weight	_____	_____	_____
Blood Pressure	___/___	___/___	___/___

YMCA of the USA
Physical Fitness Evaluation Profile

Norms—Men 46-55

Name _____ Dates: T1 _____ T2 _____ T3 _____

Rating	% ranking	Resting HR	% fat	3-min step	PWC max (kgm)	Max V̇O2 (mL/kg)	Flexibility	Bench press	Half sit-ups
Excellent	100 95 90	35 53 56	8 14 16	56 77 82	2695 1900 1660	83 55 49	26 20 19	47 33 28	78 68 61
Good	85 80 75	58 60 61	17 18 19	87 89 93	1540 1460 1385	45 43 40	18 17 16	25 22 21	57 53 52
Above average	70 65 60	63 64 65	20 21 22	95 99 101	1335 1285 1240	39 38 36	15 15 14	20 17 16	51 47 44
Average	55 50 45	66 69 70	23 23 24	103 107 111	1200 1165 1125	35 33 32	13 13 12	14 13 12	41 39 36
Below average	40 35 30	72 73 74	25 26 27	113 117 119	1085 1045 1005	31 30 29	11 11 10	11 10 9	33 32 29
Poor	25 20 15	77 78 81	28 29 30	121 124 126	960 915 865	27 26 25	9 9 8	8 6 5	25 24 21
Very poor	10 5 0	84 89 103	31 33 40	131 139 159	815 710 505	24 20 13	6 4 1	2 1 0	16 11 6

Actual Scores   T1   _____ _____ _____ _____ _____ _____ _____ _____

T2   _____ _____ _____ _____ _____ _____ _____ _____

T3   _____ _____ _____ _____ _____ _____ _____ _____

	T1	T2	T3

Actual Weight   _____ _____ _____

Target Weight   _____ _____ _____

Blood Pressure   ___/___   ___/___   ___/___

YMCA of the USA
Physical Fitness Evaluation Profile

Norms—Men 56-65

Name _____ Dates: T1 _____ T2 _____ T3 _____

Rating	% ranking	Resting HR	% fat	3-min step	PWC max (kgm)	Max V̇O2 (mL/kg)	Flexibility	Bench press	Half sit-ups
Excellent	100	42	11	60	2125	65	24	41	77
	95	52	16	71	1690	50	19	28	63
	90	56	17	77	1490	43	17	24	56
Good	85	59	19	86	1400	40	16	21	53
	80	60	20	91	1325	38	15	20	49
	75	61	21	94	1260	37	15	17	48
Above average	70	63	22	97	1200	35	13	14	46
	65	64	23	99	1150	34	13	13	43
	60	65	23	100	1105	33	13	12	41
Average	55	68	24	103	1060	32	11	11	39
	50	69	25	105	1020	31	11	10	36
	45	71	25	109	980	30	11	9	33
Below average	40	72	26	111	940	28	9	8	32
	35	73	27	115	900	27	9	6	31
	30	75	27	117	865	26	9	5	28
Poor	25	76	28	119	835	25	8	4	25
	20	77	29	123	795	23	7	3	24
	15	80	29	128	735	22	6	2	21
Very poor	10	84	31	131	670	21	5	1	20
	5	88	33	136	595	18	3	0	17
	0	103	40	154	475	12	1	0	5

Actual Scores T1 ____ ____ ____ ____ ____ ____ ____ ____

T2 ____ ____ ____ ____ ____ ____ ____ ____

T3 ____ ____ ____ ____ ____ ____ ____ ____

	T1	T2	T3
Actual Weight	_____	_____	_____
Target Weight	_____	_____	_____
Blood Pressure	___/___	___/___	___/___

YMCA of the USA
Physical Fitness Evaluation Profile

Norms—Men Over 65

Name _____ Dates: T1 _____ T2 _____ T3 _____

Rating	% ranking	Resting HR	% fat	3-min step	PWC max (kgm)	Max V̇O2 (mL/kg)	Flexibility	Bench press	Half sit-ups
Excellent	100 95 90	40 53 55	12 16 18	59 74 81	1915 1415 1260	53 42 38	24 19 17	36 22 20	66 55 50
Good	85 80 75	57 59 61	19 20 20	87 91 92	1170 1090 1025	34 33 32	16 15 14	16 14 12	44 40 38
Above average	70 65 60	62 63 65	21 22 22	94 97 102	1000 975 940	31 30 29	13 12 12	10 10 10	35 32 31
Average	55 50 45	66 67 69	23 24 24	104 106 110	890 855 825	28 27 26	11 10 10	8 8 7	30 27 26
Below average	40 35 30	70 71 73	25 25 26	114 116 118	795 760 725	25 24 23	9 9 8	6 5 4	24 23 22
Poor	25 20 15	74 77 79	27 28 29	121 123 126	685 650 610	22 21 20	7 7 6	3 2 2	21 19 15
Very poor	10 5 0	83 87 103	30 32 39	130 136 151	570 485 400	18 16 10	4 3 0	1 0 0	12 10 5

Actual Scores T1 ____ ____ ____ ____ ____ ____ ____ ____

T2 ____ ____ ____ ____ ____ ____ ____ ____

T3 ____ ____ ____ ____ ____ ____ ____ ____

	T1	T2	T3

Actual Weight _____ _____ _____

Target Weight _____ _____ _____

Blood Pressure ___/___ ___/___ ___/___

YMCA of the USA
Physical Fitness Evaluation Profile

Norms—Women 18-25

Name _____ Dates: T1 _____ T2 _____ T3 _____

Rating	% ranking	Resting HR	% fat	3-min step	PWC max (kgm)	Max V̇O2 (mL/kg)	Flexibility	Bench press	Half sit-ups
Excellent	100	42	9	52	2460	95	29	66	91
	95	55	15	75	1690	69	24	49	76
	90	57	17	81	1470	59	24	42	68
Good	85	59	18	85	1345	56	22	38	64
	80	61	19	89	1270	52	22	34	61
	75	63	19	93	1200	50	22	30	58
Above average	70	64	20	96	1150	47	21	28	57
	65	65	21	98	1105	45	20	26	54
	60	67	21	102	1055	44	20	25	51
Average	55	68	22	104	1025	42	19	22	48
	50	69	23	108	990	40	19	21	44
	45	71	23	110	955	39	19	20	41
Below average	40	72	24	113	925	38	18	18	38
	35	73	25	116	885	37	18	17	37
	30	76	26	120	850	35	17	16	34
Poor	25	77	27	122	815	33	16	13	33
	20	80	29	126	775	32	16	12	32
	15	81	30	131	720	30	16	9	28
Very poor	10	84	32	135	665	27	14	6	25
	5	88	35	143	575	24	12	2	24
	0	104	43	169	500	15	7	0	11

Actual Scores   T1 _____ _____ _____ _____ _____ _____ _____ _____

T2 _____ _____ _____ _____ _____ _____ _____ _____

T3 _____ _____ _____ _____ _____ _____ _____ _____

	T1	T2	T3
Actual Weight	_____	_____	_____
Target Weight	_____	_____	_____
Blood Pressure	___/___	___/___	___/___

YMCA of the USA
Physical Fitness Evaluation Profile

Norms—Women 26-35

Name _____ Dates: T1 _____ T2 _____ T3 _____

Rating	% ranking	Resting HR	% fat	3-min step	PWC max (kgm)	Max V̇O2 (mL/kg)	Flexibility	Bench press	Half sit-ups
Excellent	100 95 90	39 54 57	7 15 16	58 74 80	2435 1620 1425	95 65 58	28 24 23	62 46 40	70 60 54
Good	85 80 75	60 61 62	18 19 20	85 89 92	1325 1245 1185	53 51 48	22 21 21	34 32 29	50 46 44
Above average	70 65 60	64 65 66	21 21 22	95 98 101	1125 1085 1045	45 44 43	20 20 20	28 25 24	41 40 37
Average	55 50 45	68 69 70	23 24 25	104 107 110	1005 965 930	41 40 37	19 19 18	22 21 18	36 34 33
Below average	40 35 30	72 73 74	26 27 28	113 116 119	895 860 825	36 35 34	17 17 16	17 16 14	32 30 28
Poor	25 20 15	77 78 81	29 30 32	122 126 129	785 745 700	32 30 28	15 15 14	13 12 9	26 24 22
Very poor	10 5 0	84 88 102	34 37 46	134 141 171	640 555 450	25 22 14	13 12 5	6 2 0	20 17 7

Actual Scores T1 ____ ____ ____ ____ ____ ____ ____ ____

T2 ____ ____ ____ ____ ____ ____ ____ ____

T3 ____ ____ ____ ____ ____ ____ ____ ____

	T1	T2	T3
Actual Weight	_____	_____	_____
Target Weight	_____	_____	_____
Blood Pressure	___/___	___/___	___/___

YMCA of the USA
Physical Fitness Evaluation Profile

Norms—Women 36-45

Name _____ Dates: T1 _____ T2 _____ T3 _____

Rating	% ranking	Resting HR	% fat	3-min step	PWC max (kgm)	Max V̇O2 (mL/kg)	Flexibility	Bench press	Half sit-ups
Excellent	100 95 90	40 55 58	9 16 18	51 77 84	1880 1435 1260	75 56 50	28 23 22	57 41 33	74 60 54
Good	85 80 75	61 62 63	19 21 22	89 92 96	1185 1120 1065	46 44 42	21 21 20	30 28 26	48 44 42
Above average	70 65 60	65 66 67	23 24 25	100 102 104	1025 985 945	41 38 37	19 19 18	24 22 21	38 36 35
Average	55 50 45	69 70 71	26 27 28	107 109 112	910 870 835	36 34 33	17 17 17	20 17 16	32 31 30
Below average	40 35 30	72 74 75	29 30 31	115 118 120	805 775 745	32 30 29	16 16 15	14 13 12	28 24 23
Poor	25 20 15	77 78 81	32 33 35	124 128 132	710 680 640	28 26 25	14 14 13	10 8 6	22 20 19
Very poor	10 5 0	83 87 102	37 40 47	137 142 169	580 500 400	24 20 12	12 10 4	4 1 0	16 14 4

Actual Scores   T1   ____ ____ ____ ____ ____ ____ ____ ____

T2   ____ ____ ____ ____ ____ ____ ____ ____

T3   ____ ____ ____ ____ ____ ____ ____ ____

	T1	T2	T3
Actual Weight	_____	_____	_____
Target Weight	_____	_____	_____
Blood Pressure	___/___	___/___	___/___

YMCA of the USA
Physical Fitness Evaluation Profile

Norms—Women 46-55

Name _____ Dates: T1 _____ T2 _____ T3 _____

Rating	% ranking	Resting HR	% fat	3-min step	PWC max (kgm)	Max V̇O2 (mL/kg)	Flexibility	Bench press	Half sit-ups
Excellent	100 95 90	43 56 58	12 19 21	63 85 91	1845 1305 1160	72 51 45	27 22 21	50 33 29	73 57 48
Good	85 80 75	61 62 64	23 24 25	95 98 101	1055 1000 955	41 39 36	20 20 19	24 22 20	44 40 37
Above average	70 65 60	65 68 69	26 27 28	104 107 110	920 885 845	35 34 32	18 18 17	18 16 14	36 35 33
Average	55 50 45	70 71 72	29 30 30	113 115 118	810 770 740	31 30 29	16 16 16	13 12 10	32 31 30
Below average	40 35 30	73 74 76	31 32 33	120 121 124	715 685 655	28 27 26	14 14 14	9 8 7	28 27 25
Poor	25 20 15	77 80 82	34 35 37	126 128 132	625 590 550	25 23 22	13 12 12	6 5 2	23 21 19
Very poor	10 5 0	85 89 104	39 41 50	137 143 171	505 440 350	20 18 11	10 8 3	1 0 0	13 9 2

Actual Scores T1 ____ ____ ____ ____ ____ ____ ____ ____

T2 ____ ____ ____ ____ ____ ____ ____ ____

T3 ____ ____ ____ ____ ____ ____ ____ ____

	T1	T2	T3
Actual Weight	_____	_____	_____
Target Weight	_____	_____	_____
Blood Pressure	___/___	___/___	___/___

YMCA of the USA
Physical Fitness Evaluation Profile

Norms—Women 56-65

Name _____ Dates: T1 _____ T2 _____ T3 _____

Rating	% ranking	Resting HR	% fat	3-min step	PWC max (kgm)	Max VO2 (mL/kg)	Flexibility	Bench press	Half sit-ups
Excellent	100 95 90	42 56 59	12 19 22	60 83 92	1530 1235 1030	58 44 40	26 21 20	42 29 24	63 55 44
Good	85 80 75	61 63 64	24 25 26	97 100 103	975 910 850	36 35 33	19 19 18	21 20 17	42 38 35
Above average	70 65 60	65 67 68	27 28 29	106 109 111	810 770 740	32 31 30	17 17 16	14 13 12	32 30 27
Average	55 50 45	69 71 72	30 31 32	113 116 118	715 690 660	28 27 26	15 15 15	10 9 8	25 24 23
Below average	40 35 30	73 75 77	33 34 35	119 123 127	635 605 580	25 24 23	14 13 13	6 5 5	22 20 18
Poor	25 20 15	79 80 81	36 37 38	129 131 135	550 525 500	22 20 19	12 11 10	4 3 2	15 12 11
Very poor	10 5 0	84 88 103	39 41 49	141 147 174	440 380 300	18 15 10	9 7 2	1 0 0	8 7 1

Actual Scores   T1   ____ ____ ____ ____ ____ ____ ____ ____

T2   ____ ____ ____ ____ ____ ____ ____ ____

T3   ____ ____ ____ ____ ____ ____ ____ ____

                 T1   T2   T3

Actual Weight   _____ _____ _____

Target Weight   _____ _____ _____

Blood Pressure   ___/___ ___/___ ___/___

YMCA of the USA
Physical Fitness Evaluation Profile

Norms—Women Over 65

Name _____ Dates: T1 _____ T2 _____ T3 _____

Rating	% ranking	Resting HR	% fat	3-min step	PWC max (kgm)	Max V̇O2 (mL/kg)	Flexibility	Bench press	Half sit-ups
Excellent	100 95 90	49 56 59	11 18 20	70 85 92	1290 1055 835	55 48 34	26 22 20	30 22 18	54 41 34
Good	85 80 75	60 63 64	22 24 25	96 98 101	740 675 650	31 30 29	19 18 18	16 14 12	33 32 31
Above average	70 65 60	66 67 68	26 27 28	104 108 111	630 610 585	28 27 26	17 17 17	10 9 8	29 28 26
Average	55 50 45	70 71 72	29 30 31	116 120 121	565 545 525	25 24 23	16 15 15	7 6 5	25 22 21
Below average	40 35 30	73 75 76	32 33 34	123 125 126	505 490 470	22 21 20	14 13 13	4 3 3	20 18 16
Poor	25 20 15	79 80 83	35 36 37	128 129 133	445 420 395	19 18 17	12 11 10	2 1 0	13 11 10
Very poor	10 5 0	86 91 97	38 40 45	135 145 155	370 350 270	16 14 10	9 7 1	0 0 0	9 8 0

Actual Scores   T1   ____ ____ ____ ____ ____ ____ ____ ____

T2   ____ ____ ____ ____ ____ ____ ____ ____

T3   ____ ____ ____ ____ ____ ____ ____ ____

	T1	T2	T3
Actual Weight	_____	_____	_____
Target Weight	_____	_____	_____
Blood Pressure	___/___	___/___	___/___

YMCA of the USA
Body Composition Profile

Norms—Men 18-25

Name _____ Dates: T1 _____ T2 _____ T3 _____

Rating	% ranking	% fat	Chest (mm)	Abdomen (mm)	Ilium (mm)	Axilla (mm)	Tricep (mm)	Back (mm)	Thigh (mm)
Very lean	100	3	1	3	4	1	2	3	1
	95	5	3	7	5	4	4	6	6
	90	7	4	8	8	5	5	7	7
Lean	85	8	5	11	9	6	6	8	8
	80	9	6	12	10	7	7	9	9
	75	10	6	13	11	8	8	9	10
Leaner than average	70	11	7	14	12	9	9	10	11
	65	11	7	15	13	9	9	10	12
	60	12	8	16	14	10	10	11	12
Average	55	13	9	17	16	11	11	12	13
	50	14	9	19	17	12	11	12	14
	45	15	10	20	18	13	11	13	14
Fatter than average	40	16	11	21	20	14	12	14	15
	35	17	12	24	21	15	12	14	16
	30	18	13	25	22	16	13	15	17
Fat	25	19	14	27	24	17	14	16	18
	20	20	15	29	26	18	15	17	19
	15	21	17	33	29	19	16	18	20
Over fat	10	23	19	36	33	23	18	20	22
	5	27	23	43	38	27	20	24	26
	0	35	34	56	51	38	29	36	37

Actual Scores T1 ____ ____ ____ ____ ____ ____ ____ ____

T2 ____ ____ ____ ____ ____ ____ ____ ____

T3 ____ ____ ____ ____ ____ ____ ____ ____

YMCA of the USA
Body Composition Profile

Norms—Men 26-35

Name _____ Dates: T1 _____ T2 _____ T3 _____

Rating	% ranking	% fat	Chest (mm)	Abdomen (mm)	Ilium (mm)	Axilla (mm)	Tricep (mm)	Back (mm)	Thigh (mm)
Very lean	100	4	1	4	2	1	2	1	1
	95	8	4	9	7	6	4	7	6
	90	10	5	12	10	7	6	8	8
Lean	85	11	6	14	11	8	7	9	9
	80	12	7	16	12	9	8	10	10
	75	13	8	17	14	10	8	11	11
Leaner than average	70	14	9	20	15	11	9	12	12
	65	15	10	21	16	12	10	13	13
	60	16	11	22	19	13	10	13	14
Average	55	17	12	24	20	14	11	14	15
	50	18	13	25	22	15	12	15	16
	45	19	14	26	23	16	13	15	17
Fatter than average	40	20	15	28	24	17	14	16	18
	35	21	16	29	27	18	14	17	19
	30	22	17	32	28	19	15	19	20
Fat	25	23	18	33	30	21	16	20	21
	20	24	19	34	32	23	17	21	22
	15	26	21	38	35	25	18	23	23
Over fat	10	27	25	41	38	27	20	25	26
	5	29	27	46	43	31	24	29	29
	0	38	39	61	57	42	33	40	41

Actual Scores T1 _____ _____ _____ _____ _____ _____ _____ _____

T2 _____ _____ _____ _____ _____ _____ _____ _____

T3 _____ _____ _____ _____ _____ _____ _____ _____

YMCA of the USA
Body Composition Profile

Norms—Men 36-45

Name _____ Dates: T1 _____ T2 _____ T3 _____

Rating	% ranking	% fat	Chest (mm)	Abdomen (mm)	Ilium (mm)	Axilla (mm)	Tricep (mm)	Back (mm)	Thigh (mm)
Very lean	100	5	1	4	3	3	2	1	1
	95	11	6	12	8	7	5	8	7
	90	13	7	14	11	9	7	9	9
Lean	85	15	8	17	13	11	8	10	10
	80	16	10	20	15	12	9	11	11
	75	17	11	21	16	13	9	12	12
Leaner than average	70	18	12	22	19	14	10	13	13
	65	19	13	24	20	15	11	14	14
	60	20	14	26	21	16	11	15	15
Average	55	21	15	28	23	17	12	16	16
	50	21	16	29	24	18	13	17	17
	45	22	17	30	25	19	13	18	18
Fatter than average	40	23	18	32	27	20	14	19	19
	35	24	19	33	28	21	15	20	20
	30	25	20	34	29	22	15	21	21
Fat	25	26	22	37	32	23	16	22	22
	20	27	23	38	33	25	17	23	23
	15	28	26	41	36	27	19	26	25
Over fat	10	29	28	45	39	29	21	29	27
	5	31	32	49	44	33	25	31	31
	0	39	45	64	58	45	33	43	42

Actual Scores   T1   ____ ____ ____ ____ ____ ____ ____ ____

T2   ____ ____ ____ ____ ____ ____ ____ ____

T3   ____ ____ ____ ____ ____ ____ ____ ____

YMCA of the USA
Body Composition Profile

Norms—Men 46-55

Name _____ Dates: T1 _____ T2 _____ T3 _____

Rating	% ranking	% fat	Chest (mm)	Abdomen (mm)	Ilium (mm)	Axilla (mm)	Tricep (mm)	Back (mm)	Thigh (mm)
Very lean	100	8	2	4	4	5	3	3	1
	95	14	6	13	9	7	5	8	7
	90	16	7	17	12	10	6	10	9
Lean	85	17	9	20	13	11	7	11	10
	80	18	10	21	14	13	8	12	11
	75	19	11	22	17	14	9	13	12
Leaner than average	70	20	13	25	18	15	10	14	13
	65	21	14	26	20	16	11	15	14
	60	22	15	28	21	17	11	16	14
Average	55	23	17	29	22	18	12	17	15
	50	23	18	30	24	19	13	18	16
	45	24	19	32	25	21	13	19	17
Fatter than average	40	25	20	33	26	22	14	20	18
	35	26	21	34	28	23	15	21	19
	30	27	22	36	29	24	15	22	20
Fat	25	28	23	38	30	25	16	24	21
	20	29	26	40	33	27	17	25	22
	15	30	27	44	36	29	19	26	23
Over fat	10	31	30	46	38	31	20	30	27
	5	33	35	50	42	35	23	34	31
	0	40	46	65	56	46	32	46	42

Actual Scores T1 _____ _____ _____ _____ _____ _____ _____ _____

T2 _____ _____ _____ _____ _____ _____ _____ _____

T3 _____ _____ _____ _____ _____ _____ _____ _____

YMCA of the USA
Body Composition Profile

Norms—Men 56-65

Name _____ Dates: T1 _____ T2 _____ T3 _____

Rating	% ranking	% fat	Chest (mm)	Abdomen (mm)	Ilium (mm)	Axilla (mm)	Tricep (mm)	Back (mm)	Thigh (mm)
Very lean	100 95 90	11 16 17	2 7 10	5 14 16	4 9 12	4 9 12	4 6 7	4 9 10	2 7 8
Lean	85 80 75	19 20 21	11 12 14	19 21 22	13 14 16	13 14 15	8 9 10	12 13 14	9 10 11
Leaner than average	70 65 60	22 23 23	15 16 17	23 24 26	17 18 20	16 17 18	11 11 12	15 16 17	12 13 14
Average	55 50 45	24 25 25	18 19 20	27 28 30	21 22 23	19 20 21	13 13 14	18 19 20	15 16 17
Fatter than average	40 35 30	26 27 27	21 22 23	31 32 34	24 25 26	22 23 24	15 15 16	21 22 23	18 18 19
Fat	25 20 15	28 29 29	24 27 30	36 38 40	28 30 32	25 26 29	17 18 20	25 26 27	20 21 23
Over fat	10 5 0	31 33 40	32 36 47	44 48 62	34 40 52	30 34 44	21 24 31	31 34 46	27 29 41

Actual Scores   T1   ____   ____   ____   ____   ____   ____   ____   ____

T2   ____   ____   ____   ____   ____   ____   ____   ____

T3   ____   ____   ____   ____   ____   ____   ____   ____

YMCA of the USA
Body Composition Profile

Norms—Men Over 65

Name _____ Dates: T1 _____ T2 _____ T3 _____

Rating	% ranking	% fat	Chest (mm)	Abdomen (mm)	Ilium (mm)	Axilla (mm)	Tricep (mm)	Back (mm)	Thigh (mm)
Very lean	100	12	3	4	4	5	5	6	4
	95	16	6	13	8	9	6	9	7
	90	18	9	15	9	11	7	10	9
Lean	85	19	10	17	10	12	8	11	10
	80	20	12	18	12	13	9	12	11
	75	20	13	19	13	14	9	13	11
Leaner than average	70	21	14	20	14	15	10	15	12
	65	22	15	21	16	16	11	16	13
	60	22	16	22	17	17	11	16	13
Average	55	23	17	23	18	18	12	17	14
	50	24	18	25	19	19	12	18	15
	45	24	19	26	20	20	13	19	15
Fatter than average	40	25	20	27	21	21	13	20	16
	35	25	21	29	22	22	14	21	17
	30	26	22	30	24	23	14	22	17
Fat	25	27	24	31	25	24	15	23	18
	20	28	25	33	26	25	15	24	19
	15	29	26	35	28	27	16	25	21
Over fat	10	30	29	38	30	29	17	27	23
	5	32	33	43	34	33	19	29	27
	0	39	44	56	45	39	25	38	31

Actual Scores T1 _____ _____ _____ _____ _____ _____ _____ _____

T2 _____ _____ _____ _____ _____ _____ _____ _____

T3 _____ _____ _____ _____ _____ _____ _____ _____

YMCA of the USA
Body Composition Profile

Norms—Women 18-25

Name _____ Dates: T1 _____ T2 _____ T3 _____

Rating	% ranking	% fat	Chest (mm)	Abdomen (mm)	Ilium (mm)	Axilla (mm)	Tricep (mm)	Back (mm)	Thigh (mm)
Very lean	100	9	1	5	4	2	4	3	3
	95	15	4	9	6	6	9	7	13
	90	17	6	10	8	7	11	8	16
Lean	85	18	7	11	9	8	12	9	18
	80	19	8	13	10	9	13	10	19
	75	19	9	14	12	9	13	10	20
Leaner than average	70	20	10	15	13	10	14	11	21
	65	21	10	16	14	11	15	11	22
	60	21	11	17	15	11	15	12	23
Average	55	22	12	18	16	12	16	13	24
	50	23	12	19	17	13	17	13	25
	45	23	13	20	18	13	18	14	26
Fatter than average	40	24	14	21	19	14	19	15	27
	35	25	15	22	20	15	20	15	28
	30	26	16	23	21	15	21	16	29
Fat	25	27	17	25	22	16	22	17	30
	20	29	18	27	25	18	23	18	33
	15	30	20	29	26	20	25	20	36
Over fat	10	32	22	31	30	22	27	22	38
	5	35	24	37	34	26	31	26	42
	0	43	34	49	47	35	41	36	55

Actual Scores T1 _____ _____ _____ _____ _____ _____ _____ _____

T2 _____ _____ _____ _____ _____ _____ _____ _____

T3 _____ _____ _____ _____ _____ _____ _____ _____

YMCA of the USA
Body Composition Profile

Norms—Women 26-35

Name _____ Dates: T1 _____ T2 _____ T3 _____

Rating	% ranking	% fat	Chest (mm)	Abdomen (mm)	Ilium (mm)	Axilla (mm)	Tricep (mm)	Back (mm)	Thigh (mm)
Very lean	100	7	1	3	2	2	2	2	1
	95	15	4	7	6	5	9	6	14
	90	16	5	9	7	7	10	7	17
Lean	85	18	6	11	8	8	11	8	18
	80	19	7	12	10	9	12	9	21
	75	20	8	13	11	9	13	9	22
Leaner than average	70	21	9	15	12	10	14	10	23
	65	21	10	16	13	11	15	11	24
	60	22	11	17	14	11	16	12	25
Average	55	23	12	19	15	12	17	13	26
	50	24	12	20	16	13	18	14	27
	45	25	13	21	18	14	19	15	29
Fatter than average	40	26	14	23	19	15	20	16	30
	35	27	15	24	20	16	21	17	31
	30	28	16	25	22	17	22	18	32
Fat	25	29	17	27	24	18	23	19	34
	20	30	19	29	26	19	25	20	35
	15	32	21	32	28	21	26	21	38
Over fat	10	34	23	35	32	23	29	25	41
	5	37	27	40	36	27	31	29	46
	0	46	36	54	50	38	42	40	59

Actual Scores   T1   _____ _____ _____ _____ _____ _____ _____ _____

T2   _____ _____ _____ _____ _____ _____ _____ _____

T3   _____ _____ _____ _____ _____ _____ _____ _____

YMCA of the USA
Body Composition Profile

Norms—Women 36-45

Name _____ Dates: T1 _____ T2 _____ T3 _____

Rating	% ranking	% fat	Chest (mm)	Abdomen (mm)	Ilium (mm)	Axilla (mm)	Tricep (mm)	Back (mm)	Thigh (mm)
Very lean	100	9	2	3	2	3	4	1	3
	95	16	4	8	6	5	10	6	16
	90	18	6	11	8	7	12	8	18
Lean	85	19	7	13	10	8	13	9	20
	80	21	8	15	11	9	14	10	22
	75	22	9	16	12	10	16	11	24
Leaner than average	70	23	10	19	14	11	17	12	25
	65	24	11	20	15	12	18	13	26
	60	25	12	21	16	13	19	14	28
Average	55	26	13	23	18	14	20	15	29
	50	27	14	24	19	15	21	16	30
	45	28	15	25	20	16	22	17	32
Fatter than average	40	29	16	27	22	17	23	18	33
	35	30	17	28	23	18	24	19	34
	30	31	18	29	24	19	25	21	36
Fat	25	32	20	32	27	21	26	22	37
	20	33	22	33	30	23	28	23	40
	15	35	24	36	32	25	29	26	42
Over fat	10	37	26	40	35	27	32	29	46
	5	40	30	44	40	31	36	34	52
	0	47	40	60	53	41	46	44	65

Actual Scores   T1   ____ ____ ____ ____ ____ ____ ____ ____

T2   ____ ____ ____ ____ ____ ____ ____ ____

T3   ____ ____ ____ ____ ____ ____ ____ ____

YMCA of the USA
Body Composition Profile

Norms—Women 46-55

Name _____ Dates: T1 _____ T2 _____ T3 _____

Rating	% ranking	% fat	Chest (mm)	Abdomen (mm)	Ilium (mm)	Axilla (mm)	Tricep (mm)	Back (mm)	Thigh (mm)
Very lean	100	12	2	5	1	4	8	3	5
	95	19	4	11	7	8	12	8	18
	90	21	6	15	9	10	14	9	19
Lean	85	23	8	18	11	11	16	10	22
	80	24	10	19	13	12	17	12	24
	75	25	11	21	14	14	18	13	26
Leaner than average	70	26	12	23	17	15	19	14	27
	65	27	13	25	18	16	20	15	28
	60	28	14	26	19	17	21	16	30
Average	55	29	15	27	21	18	22	17	31
	50	30	16	29	22	19	23	18	32
	45	30	17	30	23	20	24	19	34
Fatter than average	40	31	18	31	25	21	25	20	35
	35	32	19	33	26	22	26	21	36
	30	33	20	35	27	23	27	22	38
Fat	25	34	23	37	29	24	29	24	40
	20	35	24	39	31	25	30	26	42
	15	37	27	42	34	26	32	28	44
Over fat	10	39	30	45	37	30	34	30	47
	5	41	34	50	42	32	38	34	52
	0	50	44	64	56	43	49	46	65

Actual Scores T1 _____ _____ _____ _____ _____ _____ _____ _____

T2 _____ _____ _____ _____ _____ _____ _____ _____

T3 _____ _____ _____ _____ _____ _____ _____ _____

YMCA of the USA
Body Composition Profile

Norms—Women 56-65

Name _____ Dates: T1 _____ T2 _____ T3 _____

Rating	% ranking	% fat	Chest (mm)	Abdomen (mm)	Ilium (mm)	Axilla (mm)	Tricep (mm)	Back (mm)	Thigh (mm)
Very lean	100	12	3	2	3	4	5	4	5
	95	19	4	12	8	8	11	9	13
	90	22	7	16	11	11	14	11	18
Lean	85	24	8	20	12	12	16	12	21
	80	25	11	22	13	14	17	13	25
	75	26	12	24	16	15	18	14	26
Leaner than average	70	27	13	26	17	16	19	15	27
	65	28	15	28	19	18	21	15	29
	60	29	16	30	20	19	22	16	30
Average	55	30	17	31	21	20	23	17	31
	50	31	19	32	23	20	24	18	33
	45	32	20	34	24	21	25	19	34
Fatter than average	40	33	21	35	25	22	26	20	37
	35	34	23	36	26	24	27	21	38
	30	35	24	38	28	25	28	23	39
Fat	25	36	25	39	29	26	29	25	40
	20	37	27	42	32	28	30	26	42
	15	38	28	43	35	29	31	27	45
Over fat	10	39	31	46	37	30	34	29	47
	5	41	32	51	41	34	38	33	53
	0	49	44	64	56	43	49	44	65

Actual Scores   T1   _____ _____ _____ _____ _____ _____ _____ _____

T2   _____ _____ _____ _____ _____ _____ _____ _____

T3   _____ _____ _____ _____ _____ _____ _____ _____

YMCA of the USA
Body Composition Profile

Norms—Women Over 65

Name _____ Dates: T1 _____ T2 _____ T3 _____

Rating	% ranking	% fat	Chest (mm)	Abdomen (mm)	Ilium (mm)	Axilla (mm)	Tricep (mm)	Back (mm)	Thigh (mm)
Very lean	100	11	3	4	4	5	5	5	6
	95	18	5	12	6	7	10	7	12
	90	20	7	16	9	10	12	8	17
Lean	85	22	9	20	10	11	14	10	20
	80	24	10	21	12	12	16	11	22
	75	25	11	24	14	13	17	12	24
Leaner than average	70	26	13	25	16	14	18	13	25
	65	27	15	26	17	15	19	14	27
	60	28	16	27	18	18	20	15	28
Average	55	29	17	29	20	19	21	16	31
	50	30	18	30	21	20	22	17	32
	45	31	19	32	22	21	22	18	33
Fatter than average	40	32	20	34	23	22	23	18	35
	35	33	21	36	25	23	24	19	36
	30	34	22	37	26	24	26	20	37
Fat	25	35	23	38	29	25	27	22	39
	20	36	24	41	30	26	28	24	42
	15	37	27	44	32	27	29	25	45
Over fat	10	38	28	46	36	31	30	26	48
	5	40	33	53	38	35	34	32	52
	0	45	40	65	51	42	45	40	63

Actual Scores   T1   _____ _____ _____ _____ _____ _____ _____ _____

T2   _____ _____ _____ _____ _____ _____ _____ _____

T3   _____ _____ _____ _____ _____ _____ _____ _____

Your Guide to YMCA Fitness Analyst Release 1.0

I. Introduction

A. What Is YMCA Fitness Analyst?

YMCA Fitness Analyst is a powerful software package that gives you the very latest in fitness research in a practical and simple format. The software divides fitness program development into three logical parts—**assessment, feedback, and prescription**—so it's very easy for you, as a YMCA fitness professional, to develop and manage efficient, successful programs for your members.

YMCA Fitness Analyst gives you important resources at your fingertips for assessing a member's health and fitness status, including updated Y norms, important new Health Standards, and medical screening tools to uncover risk factors.

To provide feedback to members on their fitness status, you can use *YMCA Fitness Analyst* to generate a wide range of customized reports. You also can choose from an extensive library of ready-to-print health education reports.

Once you have determined a member's fitness status and have worked with the member to set goals, you can use the powerful exercise prescription capabilities of *YMCA Fitness Analyst* to create a customized fitness improvement program—one that will include illustrations and descriptions of exercises as well as workout schedules.

With its full complement of assessment, feedback, and prescription capabilities, plus a convenient and practical set of administrative tools, *YMCA Fitness Analyst* delivers professional management for your Y's fitness improvement programs.

B. Benefits of YMCA Fitness Analyst

YMCA administrators, instructors, and members all benefit from the powerful features of *YMCA Fitness Analyst*:

Administrators

- Consistent administration of testing by instructors
- Quality control in record keeping and reporting
- Legal protection by screening high-risk participants
- Visible benefits to members

Instructors
- Assessment of members' health and fitness status
- Feedback to members in the form of personal reports
- Individualized prescription and program development to help members reach their fitness goals

Members
- Personal progress checks
- Access to YMCA course schedules
- Health and fitness education reports

II. Standard and Comprehensive Editions

YMCA Fitness Analyst comes in two editions: the Standard Edition (Item 0-7360-2210-4, $495) and the Comprehensive Edition (Item 0-7360-2214-7, $695).

The Standard Edition of *YMCA Fitness Analyst* was developed for *adult* health and fitness program management, with comprehensive assessment and reporting features and tools for developing individualized exercise prescriptions. The Comprehensive Edition includes not only all features of the Standard Edition, but also *youth* fitness assessment and other features described in this section.

Features preceded by a check (√) are those that appear in the *YMCA Fitness Analyst* **for the first time anywhere!**

A. Features in Both Editions

Member Information

Record personal and contact information as well as emergency and physician contacts for each Y member and program participant.

Medical Status

Included on this page are two medical screening tools, the Canadian PAR-Q and the √ Medical/Health Questionnaire developed specifically for *YMCA Fitness Analyst*.

Fitness Assessment

You can use two fitness testing protocols: (1) the YMCA Adult Fitness Test Battery and (2) the Human Kinetics (HK) Adult Fitness Test Battery. You also can create your own fitness test protocol using tests from the YMCA and HK fitness test batteries. √ Health standards are included in the software for the YMCA Adult Fitness Test. These standards are the *first* to be developed for adults. They indicate the minimal levels of fitness necessary for individuals to maintain good health and reduce their risk of developing heart disease and similar illnesses. Printed reports also provide educational materials to give to members.

Lifestyle Assessment Questionnaires

√ Two lifestyle assessment questionnaires (LAQs) are available, the YMCA Health Check and the YMCA LAQ, both developed specifically for the *Fitness Analyst*. Use the LAQs to help your members and program participants understand their state of health or risk for future medical problems. Follow-up reports based on an individual's responses are available to help members make appropriate choices in their lifestyle and dietary habits.

Health and Fitness Education Reports

√ Nineteen health and fitness education reports provide solid information on a variety of topics such as exercise and aging, body composition, flexibility, exercise and psychological health, and more. These are ready to print out and give to members.

Blood Pressure

Monitor and chart blood pressure data over time for your members.

Body Circumferences

Track changes in body size over time for weight loss or to monitor increasing muscle strength and size.

Weight Log

Enter weight changes over time.

Cardio Programming

Enter and print aerobic exercise programs. Create individualized programs for your members.

Strength Programming

Develop and print strength and conditioning programs. Online illustrations are included for all exercises. Create individualized programs for your members.

Y Course Schedule

Enter your fitness classes and educational programs into one database, then choose and print specific classes and programs for a Y member or a group. It's another great way to use the software to individualize your interaction with members.

B. Additional Features in the Comprehensive Edition

The Comprehensive Edition includes everything contained in the Standard Edition plus the following features.

Youth Fitness Assessment Tests

Two fitness assessment tests for youth are included in the Comprehensive Edition: The YMCA Youth Fitness Test Battery and the √ Human Kinetics (HK) Youth Fitness Test Battery. Like the adult tests, you can create your own fitness test protocol using tests from the YMCA and HK test batteries. √ Included in the YMCA Youth Fitness Test Battery is an additional method for calculating body composition—Body Mass Index. Results are given using the Y's youth classifications: Good, Borderline, and Needs Work.

Health Risk Assessments

The Comprehensive Edition contains nine health risk assessments (HRAs) covering a variety of health topics such as lifestyle assessment, general well-being, osteoporosis, heart risk, and diabetes.

Health and Fitness Goals

Record up to three goals for each individual.

Energy Expenditure

Track total caloric expenditure to assist in weight management programs.

Aerobic Log

Enter aerobic activities, create aerobic conditioning programs, and record the distance or duration of an activity and the number of calories used during the activity.

Total Activity Log

This log lets you keep track of all activities from workouts to household and gardening activities.

Staff Scheduling

This complete scheduling system will keep a list of appointments and tasks for your staff.

III. Assessment

A. Member Information Page

YMCA *Fitness Analyst* makes it very easy to collect and organize personal information for each member (figure 1). Collecting data on individual members is an important part of designing effective, personalized fitness improvement programs. Having the data available in such a complete and accessible format makes this software a helpful tool for organizing member information.

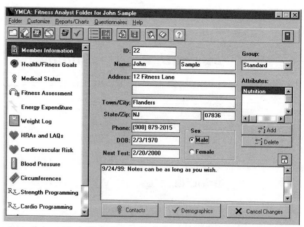

Figure 1 Member Information page.

B. Medical Status Page

The Medical Status page helps you gather information about a member's health history and current lifestyle habits in order to assess her or his readiness for both fitness testing and exercise prescription (figure 2). This capability is vital to ensure the member's safety and to protect your YMCA from liability. Included in the software are two screening tools from which you can choose the format that best suits the needs of your facility: the Canadian PAR-Q and the Medical/Health Questionnaire developed specifically for *YMCA Fitness Analyst*.

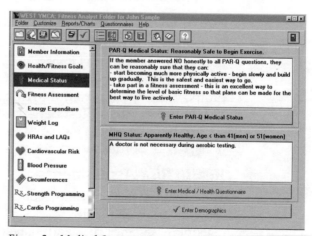

Figure 2 Medical Status page.

C. *Fitness Assessment Page*

With the availability of both the YMCA Adult Fitness Test Battery and the Human Kinetics Adult Fitness Test Battery, you can create your own fitness test protocol. The YMCA Adult Fitness Test Battery includes both the new half sit-up test and the 1997 YMCA fitness test norms.

From the Fitness Assessment page (figure 3) you can take the following actions:

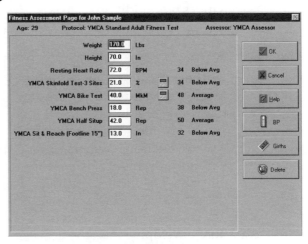

Figure 3   *Fitness Assessment page.*

• Enter fitness test results for Y members and participants

• Select a fitness protocol to meet the needs of your facility

• Create your own fitness protocol from a database of well-known fitness tests

• Establish fitness test goals for a Y member

• Track a member's progress over time through charts and graphs

• Print fitness charts and graphs

• Provide educational information to members to explain their test results using health standards and follow-up reports

D. *Health Standards*

Health standards are included in *YMCA Fitness Analyst* to aid Y staff in interpreting fitness test scores. These standards are the *first* to be developed for adults. Health standards indicate the minimal levels of fitness necessary for individuals to maintain good health and to reduce their risk of developing heart disease and other illnesses.

Norms, on the other hand, provide a comparison of an individual's results against the results of a large population sample, generally made up of people of the same age and gender. Consequently, norms are useful for individuals who want to know how they compare to others of their same age and gender.

Having both health standards and norms available to interpret fitness test results means you can provide quality feedback to your members on the state of their fitness and health.

E. *Lifestyle Assessment Questionnaires/Health Risk Assessments*

Lifestyle assessment questionnaires, or LAQs, help participants understand their state of health or risk for future medical problems. Reports are also available to help members make appropriate choices in their lifestyles and dietary habits. The Standard Edition of *YMCA Fitness Analyst* includes two LAQs—the YMCA Health Check and the YMCA Lifestyle Assessment Questionnaire (figure 4). The

Comprehensive Edition includes nine additional Health Risk Assessments, or HRAs. The YMCA LAQ is a comprehensive questionnaire that includes assessment of a person's health and fitness goals as well as lifestyle activities. This information allows you to determine whether or not an individual wishes to improve his or her health or fitness—an issue that you and the member must address before developing any physical improvement program. The YMCA Health Check, by comparison, is a briefer assessment.

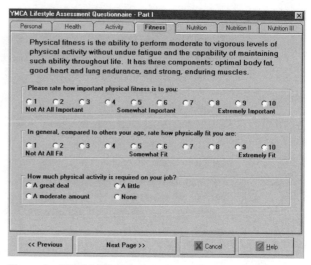

Figure 4   YMCA Lifestyle Assessment Questionnaire.

You or the members can enter responses to HRAs and LAQs directly onscreen, or you can print out the forms for members to complete. After you have entered the information, the software will use the results to produce the reports.

F. Framingham Cardiovascular Heart Disease Risk Analysis Page

The Framingham Cardiovascular Heart Disease (CHD) Risk Analysis page (figure 5) calculates a member's risk of CHD based on several factors, including smoking habits, blood pressure, and cholesterol levels. The Framingham CHD Risk Analysis is a powerful tool for helping members identify lifestyle behaviors that pose potential risks to them. As part of your facility's fitness and wellness education program, you can provide information to your members on positive lifestyle choices that will reduce their risk of CHD.

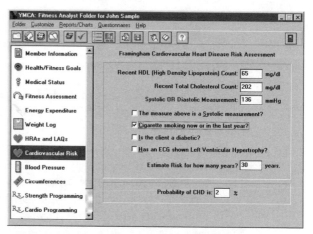

Figure 5   Framingham CHD Risk Analysis page.

IV. Feedback

YMCA Fitness Analyst can generate many reports and graphs that show individual progress and provide information on key health and fitness topics (see an example in figure 6). Members get fitness comparisons not only to established norms but also to the scientifically developed Health Standards created uniquely for the YMCA. These printouts are strong motivational tools. They can help your members gain a deeper understanding of how their fitness scores relate to good health and of the benefits of their personalized fitness program.

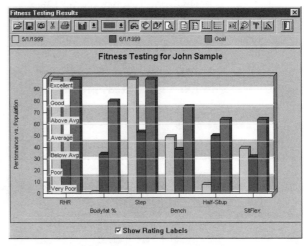

Figure 6   Fitness testing report.

A. Health and Fitness Education Reports

The following health and fitness education reports provide solid information on a variety of topics such as exercise and aging, overtraining, and body composition. These reports can be printed out and given to members. Figure 7 is a sample Health and Fitness Education Report.

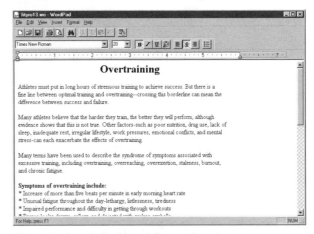

Figure 7   Sample health and fitness education report.

- Assessment Preparation
- Physical Fitness
- Cardiorespiratory Fitness
- Body Composition
- Muscular Strength and Endurance
- Flexibility
- Activity Readiness
- Selection of Aerobic Exercise Mode
- Comprehensive Fitness
- Exercise Progress/Sticking to It
- The Warm-Up and Cool-down
- The Exercise Heart Rate
- Overtraining

- Laboratory Tests for Cardiorespiratory Fitness
- Risk Factors for Heart Disease
- Weight Management
- Hydration
- Exercise and Psychological Health
- Exercise and Aging

B. Charts

As you use *YMCA Fitness Analyst*, you'll see that the information entered into the software can be used to generate and print many reports and graphs for the benefit of staff and members. These printouts are strong motivational tools that can help your members gain a deeper understanding of their current state of health and fitness and how they can gain the benefits of exercise. Figures 8 and 9 show examples of available charts; a complete list appears below.

- All Fitness Tests: Change Over Time
- All Fitness Tests: One Date
- Summary Score: Change Over Time
- Single Fitness Test Rank: Change Over Time
- Single Fitness Test Raw Score: Change Over Time
- Body Composition Pie Chart: One Date
- Body Composition: Change Over Time
- Blood Pressure: Change Over Time
- Waist-Hip Ratio: Change Over Time
- Body Circumferences: Change Over Time
- Weight: Change Over Time
- Calories Expended: Change Over Time
- Aerobic Log Over Time
- Total Activity Log

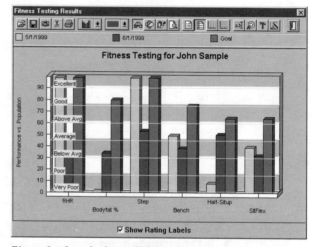

Figure 8   Sample chart: all fitness tests.

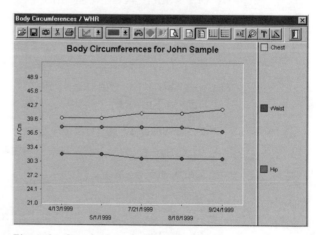

Figure 9   Sample chart: body circumferences.

C. Member Reports

The following reports contain valuable member information that is collected throughout the software. These reports assemble the information in efficient formats that are easy to review and print out for members. Figure 10 shows a typical report.

- Comprehensive Report of Findings
- Member Fitness Assessments
- Body Composition Summary
- Member Goal Report
- Medical Health Questionnaire Report
- YMCA Health Check Report
- YMCA Lifestyle Assessment Report
- Blood Pressure Log
- Framingham Risk Report
- Aerobic Prescription Report
- Aerobic Log

Figure 10   Sample report: member fitness assessment.

D. Weight Log Page

The Weight Log page provides you with an easy, convenient way to track a member's weight over time.

E. Blood Pressure Page

With the Blood Pressure page you can monitor and chart blood pressure (BP) data over time, maintain a record of resting BP, or combine resting BP measurements with exercise BP data.

F. Circumferences (Girth) Page

On this page you can track changes in body size over time as a means of measuring progress in weight loss or muscle gain programs (figure 11). A number of measurements can be taken: neck, shoulder, waist, hip, and right and left side measurements for thigh, calf, leg, and forearm. A feature of the Circumferences

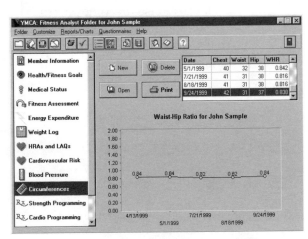

Figure 11   Circumferences (Girth) page.

(Girth) page is the automatic calculation of waist-hip ratio, a valuable predictive measure for the health implications of obesity.

V. Exercise Prescription

The powerful capabilities of the tools described in this section allow you to design personalized exercise programs based on your members' individual goals. Whether participants' goals are increased muscular strength or aerobic fitness, you can include drawings and descriptions of specific exercises within a comprehensive program. You can then use the monitoring features and other reports to track each individual's progress toward his or her fitness goals.

A. Strength Programming Page

With its extensive exercise library of drawings and descriptions, the Strength Programming page (figure 12) allows you to create complete, detailed strength training regimens for your members. You can modify the drawings and descriptions, group the exercises to focus on specific areas, print the programs, and save the programs you create.

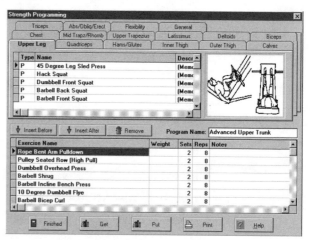

Figure 12   Strength Programming page.

B. Cardio Programming Page

Like the Strength Programming page, the Cardio Programming page (figure 13) allows you to create individual programs by extracting exercises from an extensive library. These exercises become part of an aerobic fitness program for cardiorespiratory improvement.

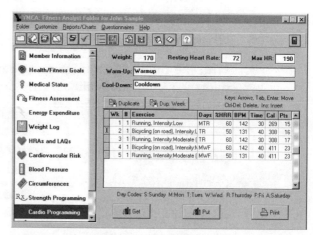

Figure 13   Cardio Programming page.

VI. Administrative Features

A. Password Security

Password security offers you complete control over sensitive information about members (figure 14). Each user is granted access at one of three levels; the access level determines the extent to which each user can view and manipulate not only member data but also other information contained within *YMCA Fitness Analyst.*

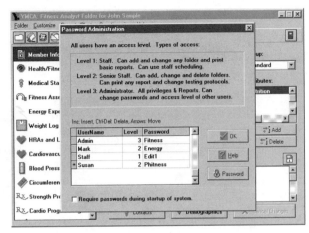

Figure 14   Password administration.

B. Program Customization

Convenient program customization allows you to specify whether certain optional features appear or not when the program is launched (figure 15). The software also allows you to export research data for later collection by the YMCA to determine future YMCA fitness norms.

Your copy of *YMCA Fitness Analyst* will be customized with the name of your facility on the Welcome screen and the title bar of each page. The

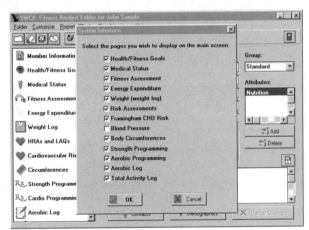

Figure 15   Program customization feature.

name, address, and phone number of your YMCA will appear on each report.

C. Group Management and Reports

The following features simplify the task of managing a member base. These features are also valuable to members because they make it easy for YMCA staff to keep in touch with them and to keep track of their status.

- Fitness Results Breakdown by Group
- Member List
- Member Mailing Labels
- Members Needing Reassessment
- Members by Attribute

D. Y Course Schedule

The Y Course Schedule is a convenient, powerful group management tool that allows you to enter fitness and educational programs into one database, and then choose and print specific classes and programs for a Y member or group (figure 16). By selecting classes and programs that would benefit members who are experiencing specific health or exercise problems, or by suggesting classes to those members who simply want to

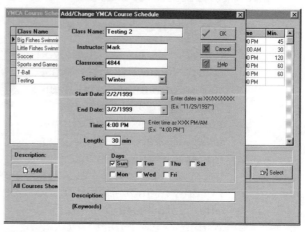

Figure 16   The Y Course Schedule.

add to their fitness regimen, you can use the Y Course Schedule as another way to individualize your interaction with members.

VII. When You Need Help

A. The Help System

YMCA Fitness Analyst includes an extensive Help system featuring thorough, easy-to-read coverage of a wide range of topics. For most questions, the answer is a keypress away.

B. User Guide

The *YMCA Fitness Analyst User Guide* includes detailed coverage of nearly every aspect of the software. It is organized into the following parts:

Part I provides an overview of *YMCA Fitness Analyst* and covers system requirements and installation procedures.

Part II discusses login procedures, the role of the software administrator, security features, and system customization.

Part III describes all the sections, or pages, of the software and explains the graphic elements on each screen (e.g., icons, pull-down menus).

Part IV includes those features that are part of both the Standard and Comprehensive editions of the software.

Part V covers features that are exclusive to the Comprehensive Edition.

Part VI provides instructions on how to produce the many available reports, charts, and graphs.

Part VII goes into greater detail on fitness testing, including how to develop custom testing protocols.

Part VIII covers backup procedures for protecting and preserving the valuable information you've collected.

Part IX details troubleshooting procedures.

C. *Customer Support*

Unlimited free technical support from the YMCA Program Store is also available for those occasions when you need additional assistance from a software specialist. Technical support is available Monday through Friday from 8 AM to 5 PM, CST, by calling 217-351-5077. You can also send e-mail to **support@hkusa.com** to get answers to questions of a less urgent nature.

> The YMCA Program Store stands behind the *YMCA Fitness Analyst* software and offers a dedicated customer support staff to answer your questions and listen to your suggestions and concerns.

VIII. System Requirements

YMCA Fitness Analyst requires a 386 or higher IBM PC or compatible, Microsoft Windows 3.1 or later (Windows 95 is recommended but not required), 6MB RAM (8MB recommended), and 20MB hard disk space.

IX. Licensing and Software Usage

1. Permitted Uses. The YMCA Program Store grants you the non-exclusive license to use this software according to the following terms. You may use the software on a single computer. If you have more than one computer on which you would like to run the software, then you must contact the YMCA Program Store to purchase additional copies. The software cannot be used in any other manner without violating this agreement.

2. Prohibited Uses. Without the express written permission of the YMCA Program Store you may not

- make the software available to any other organization, entity, or person other than yourself or your organization.
- copy, sell, sublicense, rent, lease, give, or lend copies of this software or its component parts (e.g., exercise pictures) to others.
- operate this software on more than one computer at a time.
- disassemble, decompile, reverse engineer, or make any attempt to discover the source code of this software.
- translate or create derivative works based on the software.
- modify this software or merge it with another program.

X. Ordering Information

Order Form				
Item Number	Quantity	Description	Price	Total
0-7360-2210-4		*YMCA Fitness Analyst* Standard Edition, Release 1.0	$495.00	
0-7360-2214-7		*YMCA Fitness Analyst* Comprehensive Edition, Release 1.0	$695.00	

Customization: Enter the name of your YMCA below (up to 32 characters).

_____

Send orders to:

YMCA Program Store
P.O. Box 5076
Champaign, IL 61825-5076
800-747-0089
Fax: 217-351-1549

Bill to:

Name_____

Address_____

City_____State_____

Zip_____Phone____-____-_____

Purchase Order Number_____

Ship to (if different than Bill to):

Name_____

Address_____

City_____State_____

Zip_____Phone____-____-_____

Purchase Order Number_____

Subtotal _____

IL residents add 6.25% sales tax
(personal orders only!) _____

Add postage/handling _____

Total _____

All prices subject to change.

Personal Orders and Postage/Handling

Prepayment in U.S. funds is required. Personal orders must be prepaid by check, money order, or credit card. All orders are sent via UPS. For shipping of personal orders, please include $4.75 for the first item and $1.00 for each additional item. For complete ordering information and sales terms, please see the YMCA Program Store catalog.

❏ My check or money order is enclosed.

Charge my ❏ Visa   ❏ MasterCard
❏ American Express

Acct. No. _____

Expiration Date _____

Signature _____

NOTE: We cannot process credit card orders without
your signature!

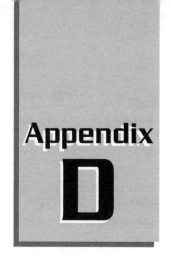

Energy Expenditure in Household, Recreational, and Sports Activities (in kcal · min⁻¹)

Appendix D

How to use: Change your body weight into kilograms (divide weight in pounds by 2.2), for example a male weighing 80 kg. Find the activity and multiply value by weight, e.g. fishing = 0.062. 0.062 × 80 = 4.96 cal/min. If done for an hour: 4.96 × 60 = 297.6 calories.

Activity	kcal·min⁻¹·kg⁻¹	Activity	kcal·min⁻¹·kg⁻¹	Activity	kcal·min⁻¹·kg⁻¹
Archery	0.065	Cooking (F)	0.045	Fishing	0.062
Badminton	0.097	Cooking (M)	0.048	Food shopping (F)	0.062
Bakery, general (F)	0.035	Cricket		Food shopping (M)	0.058
Basketball	0.138	batting	0.083	Football	0.132
Billiards	0.042	bowling	0.090	Forestry	
Bookbinding	0.038	Croquet	0.059	ax chopping, fast	0.297
Boxing		Cycling		ax chopping, slow	0.085
in ring	0.222	leisure, 5.5 mph	0.064	barking trees	0.123
sparring	0.138	leisure, 9.4 mph	0.100	carrying logs	0.186
Canoeing		racing	0.169	felling trees	0.132
leisure	0.044	Dancing		hoeing	0.091
racing	0.103	Dancing (F)		planting by hand	0.109
Card playing	0.025	aerobic, medium	0.103	sawing by hand	0.122
Carpentry, general	0.052	aerobic, intense	0.135	sawing, power	0.075
Carpet sweeping (F)	0.045	ballroom	0.051	stacking firewood	0.088
Carpet sweeping (M)	0.048	choreographed		trimming trees	0.129
Circuit training		"twist," "wiggle"	0.168	weeding	0.072
Hydra-Fitness	0.132	Digging trenches	0.145	Furriery	0.083
Universal	0.116	Drawing (standing)	0.036	Gardening	
Nautilus	0.092	Eating (sitting)	0.023	digging	0.126
Free Weights	0.086	Electrical work	0.058	hedging	0.077
Cleaning (F)	0.062	Farming		mowing	0.112
Cleaning (M)	0.058	barn cleaning	0.135	raking	0.054
Climbing hills		driving harvester	0.040	Golf	0.085
with no load	0.121	driving tractor	0.037	Gymnastics	0.066
with 5-kg load	0.129	feeding cattle	0.085	Horse grooming	0.128
with 10-kg load	0.140	feeding animals	0.065	Horse racing	
with 20-kg load	0.147	forking straw bales	0.138	galloping	0.137
Coal mining		milking by hand	0.054	trotting	0.110
drilling coal, rock	0.094	milking by machine	0.023	walking	0.041
erecting supports	0.088	shoveling grain	0.085	Ironing (F)	0.033
shoveling coal	0.108	Field hockey	0.134	Ironing (M)	0.064

Activity	kcal·min⁻¹·kg⁻¹	Activity	kcal·min⁻¹·kg⁻¹	Activity	kcal·min⁻¹·kg⁻¹
Judo	0.195	Plastering	0.078	hand rolling	0.137
Jumping rope		Printing	0.035	merchant mill	
70 per min	0.162	Racquetball	0.178	rolling	0.145
80 per min	0.164	Running, cross-country	0.163	removing slag	0.178
125 per min	0.177	Running, horizontal		tending furnace	0.126
145 per min	0.197	11 min, 30 s per mile	0.135	tipping molds	0.092
Knitting, sewing (F)	0.022	9 min per mile	0.193	Stock clerking	0.054
Knitting, sewing (M)	0.023	8 min per mile	0.208	Swimming	
Locksmithing	0.057	7 min per mile	0.228	backstroke	0.169
Lying at ease	0.022	6 min per mile	0.252	breaststroke	0.162
Machine tooling		5 min, 30 s per mile	0.289	crawl, fast	0.156
machining	0.048	Scraping paint	0.063	crawl, slow	0.128
operating lathe	0.052	Scrubbing floors (F)	0.109	sidestroke	0.122
operating punch		Scrubbing floors (M)	0.108	treading, fast	0.170
press	0.088	Shoe repair, general	0.045	treading, normal	0.062
tapping and drilling	0.065	Sitting quietly	0.021	Table tennis	0.068
welding	0.052	Skiing, hard snow		Tailoring	
working sheet		level, moderate		cutting	0.041
metal	0.048	speed	0.119	hand sewing	0.032
Marching, rapid	0.142	level, walking	0.143	machine sewing	0.045
Mopping floor (F)	0.062	uphill, maximum		pressing	0.062
Mopping floor (M)	0.058	speed	0.274	Tennis	0.109
Music playing		Skiing, soft snow		Typing	
accordion (sitting)	0.032	leisure (F)	0.111	electric	0.027
cello (sitting)	0.041	leisure (M)	0.098	manual	0.031
conducting	0.039	Skindiving, as frogman		Volleyball	0.050
drums (sitting)	0.066	considerable motion	0.276	Walking, normal pace	
flute (sitting)	0.035	moderate motion	0.206	asphalt road	0.080
horn (sitting)	0.029	Snowshoeing,		fields and hillsides	0.082
organ (sitting)	0.053	soft snow	0.166	grass track	0.081
piano (sitting)	0.040	Squash	0.212	plowed field	0.077
trumpet (standing)	0.031	Standing quietly (F)	0.025	Wallpapering	0.048
violin (sitting)	0.045	Standing quietly (M)	0.027	Watch repairing	0.025
woodwind (sitting)	0.032	Steel mill, working in		Window cleaning (F)	0.059
Painting, inside	0.034	fettling	0.089	Window cleaning (M)	0.058
Painting, outside	0.077	forging	0.100	Writing (sitting)	0.029
Planting seedlings	0.070				

Note. Data from McArdle, W.D., Katch, F.I., and Katch, V.L.: *Exercise Physiology.* Lea & Febiger, Philadelphia, 1986. Data from E.W. Bannister and S.R. Brown, The relative energy requirements of physical activity in H.B. Falls, ed., *Exercise Physiology,* Academic Press, New York, 1968; E.T. Howley and M.E. Glover, The caloric costs of running and walking one mile for men and women, *Medicine and Science in Sports* 6:235, 1974. R. Passmore and J.V.G.A. Durnin, Human energy expenditure, *Physiological Reviews,* 35:801, 1955. Symbols (M) and (F) denote experiments for males and females, respectively.

References

American College of Sports Medicine. (2000). *Guidelines for exercise testing and prescription* (6th ed.). Baltimore: Lippincott Williams & Wilkins.

American Heart Association. (1972). *Exercise testing and training of apparently healthy individuals: A handbook for physicians.* New York.

American Heart Association. (1975). *Exercise testing and training of individuals with heart disease or at high risk for its development: A handbook for physicians.* New York.

Åstrand, P.-O., & Rhyming, I. (1954). A nomogram for calculation of aerobic capacity (physical fitness) from pulse rate during submaximal work. *Journal of Applied Physiology, 7,* 218-221.

Bioelectrical Impedance Analysis in Body Composition Measurement. NIH Technol Assess Statement 1994 Dec 12-14; 1-35.

Brozek, J., Grande, F., Anderson, J.T., & Keys, A. (1963). Densitometric analysis of body composition: Revision of some quantitative assumptions. *Annals of the New York Academy of Science, 110,* 113.

Cureton, T.K., Jr. (1941). Flexibility as an aspect of physical fitness. *Research Quarterly Supplement, 12,* 388-390.

Faulkner, R.A., Sprigings, E.J., McQuarrie, A., & Bell, R.D. (1989). A partial curl-up protocol for adults based on the analysis of two procedures. *Canadian Journal of Sports & Science, 14(3),* 135-141.

Flint, M.M. (1965). An electromyographic comparison of the function of the iliacus and the rectus abdominis muscles: A preliminary report. *Journal of the American Physical Therapy Association, 45(3),* 248-253.

Godfrey, K.E., Kindig, L.E., & Windell, E.J. (1977). Electromyographic study of duration of muscle activity in sit-up variations. *Archives of Physical Medicine & Rehabilitation, 58,* 132-135.

Golding, L.A. (1988). *Differences in skinfold measurements using different calipers.* Unpublished manuscript.

Gruber, J.S., & Pollock, M.L. (1988). *Comparison of Harpenden and Lange calipers in predicting body composition.*

Halpern, A.A., & Bleck, E.E. (1979). Sit-up exercises: An electromyographic study. *Clinical Orthopaedics & Related Research, 145,* 172-178.

Jackson, A.S., & Pollock, M.L. (1978). Generalized equations for predicting body density of man. *British Journal of Nutrition, 40,* 497-504.

Jette, M., Sidney, K., & Cicutti, N. (1984). A critical analysis of sit-ups: A case for the partial curl-up as a test of abdominal muscular endurance. *Canadian Association for Health, Physical Education & Recreation, 51(1),* 4-9.

Johnson, B.L., & Nelson, J.K. (1979). *Practical measurement for evaluation in physical education.* Minneapolis: Burgess.

LaBan, M.M., Raptou, A.D., & Johnsons, E.W. (1965). Electromyographic study of function of the ilio-psoas muscle. *Archives of Physical Medicine & Rehabilitation,* Oct., 676-679.

McArdle, W.D., Katch, F.I., & Katch, V.L. (1981). *Exercise physiology*. Philadelphia: Lea & Febiger.

Reebok International, Ltd. (1991). Assessing abdominal strength: One minute curl-up test. *Reebok International, Ltd.* Instructor News. Dallas, TX: Institute for Aerobic Research.

Robertson, L.D., & Magnusdottir, H. (1987). Evaluation of criteria associated with abdominal fitness testing. *Research Quarterly for Exercise & Sport, 58(3)*, 355-359.

Scott, M.G., & French, E. (1959). *Measurement and evaluation in physical education*. Dubuque, IA: Brown.

Siri, W.E. (1956). Gross composition of the body. In J.H. Lawrence & C.A. Tobias (Eds.), *Advances in biological and medical physics* (Vol. 4) (pp. 239-280). New York: Academic Press.

Sjostrand, T. (1947). Changes in the respiratory organs of workmen at an ore melting works. *Acta Medica Scandinavica, 128* (Suppl. 196), 687-699.

Walters, E.C., & Partridge, M.J. (1956). Electromyographic study of the differential action of the abdominal muscles during exercise. *American Journal of Physical Medicine*. 259-266.

Wilmore, J.H. (1983). Body composition in sport and exercise: Directions for future research. *Medicine and Science in Sports and Exercise, 15*, 21.

YMCA of the USA. (1995). *YMCA Exercise Instructor Manual*. Champaign, IL: Human Kinetics.

Index

The italicized *t* and *f* indicate tables and figures.

Additional Resources for Your Fitness Program

See the YMCA Program Store catalog for details about these additional items for your YMCA fitness program or contact the Program Store, P.O. Box 5076, Champaign, IL 61825-5076, phone 800-747-0089. To save time, order by fax, 217-351-1549. (Please call if you are interested in receiving a free catalog.)

Fitness Program Resources

0-7360-2214-7	YMCA Fitness Analyst (Comprehensive Edition)	$695.00
0-7360-2210-4	YMCA Fitness Analyst (Standard Edition)	$495.00
0-87322-263-6	YMCA Youth Fitness Test Manual	$ 13.00
0-87322-755-7	YMCA Personal Training Instructor Manual	$ 32.00
1-887781-00-5	Get Real: A Personal Guide to Real-Life Weight Management	$ 15.95
0-7360-0146-8	YMCA/IDEA Get Real Weight Management Instructor Manual	$ 18.00
0-88011-949-7	YMCA Personal Fitness Program Manual	$ 28.00
0-7360-0186-7	Principles of YMCA Health and Fitness (Third Edition)	$ 22.00
0-87322-884-7	YMCA Exercise Instructor Manual	$ 28.00
0-7360-1030-0	Performance Aerobics, Hi/Lo Impact 40 Audio	$ 22.95
0-88011-543-2	YMCA Walk Reebok Instructor Manual	$ 49.00
0-88011-899-7	YMCA Walk Reebok Distance/Interval Training Instructor Manual	$ 16.00
0-87322-717-4	YMCA Healthy Back Program Instructor's Guide	$ 22.00
0-87322-629-1	YMCA Healthy Back Book	$ 12.95
0-87322-692-5	YMCA Healthy Back Video	$ 19.95
0-88011-967-5	Exercises for a Healthy Back Poster	$ 15.00
0-88011-966-7	Stretching Basics Poster	$ 15.00
0-88011-792-3	YMCA Fun and Fitness Activity Chart	$ 5.00
0-7360-0971-X	YMCA Fitness Assessment Guide to Setting Workloads	$ 3.00
0-7360-1011-4	YMCA Heart Rate Check Poster	$ 15.00
0-88011-942-X	Exercise for Older Adults	$ 25.00
0-88011-817-2	Guidelines for Cardiac Rehabilitation and Secondary Prevention Programs (Third Edition)	$ 35.00
0-87322-614-3	Conditioning With Physical Disabilities	$ 22.95
0-87322-392-6	Arthritis: Your Complete Exercise Guide	$ 13.95
0-87322-427-2	Diabetes: Your Complete Exercise Guide	$ 13.95

Prices shown are subject to change